Guide to Assessment Scales in
Attention-deficit/ Hyperactivity Disorder

Second Edition

Scott H. Kollins
Associate Professor
Director, Duke ADHD Program
Department of Psychiatry
Duke University Medical Center
Durham, NC

Elizabeth P. Sparrow
Clinical Neuropsychologist
Sparrow Neuropsychology, PA
Raleigh, NC

Editor
C. Keith Conners
Professor Emeritus
Duke University Medical Center
Durham, NC

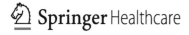 Springer Healthcare

Published by Springer Healthcare Ltd, 236 Gray's Inn Road, London, WC1X 8HB, UK

springerhealthcare.com

British Library Cataloguing-in-Publication Data.

A catalogue record for this book is available from the British Library.

ISBN 978-1-907673-15-3

Although every effort has been made to ensure that drug doses and other information are presented accurately in this publication, the ultimate responsibility rests with the prescribing physician. Neither the publisher nor the authors can be held responsible for errors or for any consequences arising from the use of the information contained herein. Any product mentioned in this publication should be used in accordance with the prescribing information prepared by the manufacturers. No claims or endorsements are made for any drug or compound at present under clinical investigation.

Project editor: Teresa Salazar
Designer: Joe Harvey
Artworker: Sissan Mollerfors
Production: Marina Maher

Contents

Biographies

Authors

Scott H. Kollins, PhD, is an Associate Professor in the Department of Psychiatry at Duke University Medical Center, North Carolina. He completed his undergraduate degree at Duke University, and earned his doctorate in clinical psychology from Auburn University. His primary research areas of expertise pertain to the psychopharmacology of stimulant drugs used to treat attention-deficit/hyperactivity disorder (ADHD) and the comorbidity of nicotine dependence and ADHD. He is an elected member of both the College on Problems of Drug Dependence and the American College of Neuropsychopharmacology. He has published more than 70 peer-reviewed scientific papers and his research has been consistently funded for over 10 years by federal and industry sources. He has 15 years of clinical experience working with ADHD individuals and their families. The ADHD Program at Duke University, which Dr Kollins directs, serves more than 150 families annually from across the US and the world.

Elizabeth P. Sparrow, PhD, is a clinical neuropsychologist in private practice in Raleigh, North Carolina. She received her doctorate in clinical psychology from Washington University in St. Louis, Missouri, with a clinical internship in neuropsychology at the University of Chicago and post-doctoral residency in pediatric neuropsychology at the Kennedy Krieger Institute and Johns Hopkins University School of Medicine. Prior to pursuing her doctorate, Dr Sparrow worked with Dr Conners in his ADHD Clinic at Duke University Medical Center. In addition to private practice, Dr Sparrow has served as a consultant to test publishers to improve assessment tools for ADHD. She has also provided consultation to the pharmaceutical industry to improve research on new compounds for ADHD, including measure selection and rater training in adult and pediatric ADHD clinical trials. Dr Sparrow has presented on ADHD and related disorders at national and international conferences, as well as providing local training seminars on identification of ADHD across the lifespan. Publications include journal articles, book chapters, and most recently, a book, *Essentials of Conners Behavior Assessments*.

Editor

C. Keith Conners is Professor Emeritus, Duke University Medical Center in Durham, North Carolina. He had an extraordinary career as an academic, clinician, researcher, lecturer, author, editor-in-chief, and administrator. Dr Conners received his PhD from Harvard University, Massachusetts. His focus on ADHD grew while working as a clinical psychiatrist and research assistant at Johns Hopkins Hospital, Maryland. Dr Conners' first task was to analyze data for a study of the effects of dexedrine on symptomatology in delinquents. When he recognized that a lot of the children underwent remarkable improvements on dexedrine and ritalin, he realized that it was a lifelong topic of study. He was also impressed by the teacher's ability to recognize dramatic changes in drug-treated children. This discovery led to his use of teacher ratings as a way of documenting drug changes. Dr Conners saw many children whose diverse pattern of symptoms interested him. Employing another symptom list already in use, he collected data on normal and clinical children, and eventually published the first version of the Parent Rating Scale. The increasing use of the rating scales eventually made his original articles among the most cited in the literature. He has written several books on attention disorders and neuropsychology, and hundreds of journal articles and book chapters based on his research regarding the effects of food additives, nutrition, stimulant drugs, diagnosis, and dimensional syndromes.

Preface

Rating scales have been an important component of both the clinical and scientific study of attention-deficit/hyperactivity disorder (ADHD) since the 1960s; and, accordingly, the number and quality of these scales has increased dramatically. The wide range of ages, covering early childhood, school ages, adolescents, and adults, requires tools with normative coverage across those periods. In addition, variations due to gender and other complicating (comorbid) disorders pose further challenges in rating scale assessment.

The available rating scales reflect considerable variation in approach. Some are focused on specific ages, some combine normative data for both genders, and others add a variety of related disorders. Some rating scales are short and simple enough that they allow frequent administrations for follow-up without significant burden on the raters, while others are more complex. Clinicians and researchers will have a wide choice in selecting the rating scale(s) that best suit the particular focus and context in which they work or study.

Rating scales are capable of facilitating clinical practice because of their ability to capture a wide variety of information in an efficient manner; and, analyze and display their results in a helpful fashion. But all rating scales should be considered as an aid to clinical assessment, never as a final method for diagnosing or making decisions without expert clinical skills. Results from rating scales are *hypotheses* to be validated within the larger framework of clinical or research investigation. They usually represent the beginning, not the end, of a clinical assessment.

Much information is to be gleaned in a *qualitative* fashion, as well as the more obvious statistical and *quantitative* information derived from scores and normative comparisons. Just as an intelligence or achievement test requires thoughtful assessment of the cultural and behavioral context in which it occurs, rating scales need sensible and informed judgment.

For example, what is to be made of the disagreement between different observers, say, a teacher and parent or between two parents? Far from being a source of error, such disagreements are useful as prompts for further investigation. As another example, the pattern of responding on a scale is itself informative, regardless of the quantitative result obtained by statistical manipulations.

Our authors of this guidebook are distinguished by long experience in both scientific and clinical aspects of ADHD. We hope that the careful scrutiny of rating scales in this book will be useful in selecting and using these scales to their best advantage.

C. Keith Conners
Professor Emeritus, Duke University Medical Center, Durham, NC

November 2010

1 Introduction to assessing ADHD

Prevalence and epidemiology

Attention-deficit/hyperactivity disorder (ADHD) is a genetically heritable, biologically driven disorder that involves developmentally inappropriate levels of inattention, hyperactivity, and impulsivity.[1] ADHD is among the most common of psychiatric disorders, affecting approximately 8% or 9% of school-aged children and 4.4–5.2% of adults in the US.[2-5] The estimated worldwide prevalence of ADHD has been reported to be 5.3%.[6] The impact of ADHD on the health care system and society is also staggering, costing tens of billions of dollars annually in addition to personal and family costs.[7]

Comorbidity and associated features

Children with ADHD are at increased risk for the development of a wide range of comorbid psychiatric conditions, including oppositional defiant disorder, conduct disorder, mood disorders, learning disabilities, and tic disorders.[8] Functionally impairing ADHD symptoms persist into adolescence and adulthood in a substantial number of cases.[9] As is the case with children, adolescents and adults with ADHD often have comorbid illness and functional impairment, including mood problems, anxiety disorders, antisocial personality disorder, and substance abuse disorders.[10] Epidemiological studies have shown that 38% of adults with ADHD meet criteria for a mood disorder, 47% of adults with ADHD meet criteria for an anxiety disorder, and 15% of adults with ADHD meet criteria for a substance use disorder – rates that are considerably higher than the general population.[4] Beyond psychiatric comorbidity, adults with ADHD also experience a range of functional impairments, including lower educational attainment, lower vocational achievement, more driving accidents, more difficulty in family and interpersonal relationships, and more legal difficulties.[11,12]

Age- and gender-based differences in ADHD

ADHD is a heterogeneous disorder both within and across gender and age groups. Although a number of factors influence prevalence rates, in children, boys are diagnosed with ADHD between three and nine times more often than girls, and diagnosed girls typically show lower ratings of core symptoms, more intellectual impairment, and higher rates of internalizing disorders.[13,14] In samples of adults, females appear to be diagnosed at comparable rates as males.[15]

With respect to diagnostic heterogeneity, it is also important to consider that ADHD symptoms recognized in the *Diagnostic and Statistical Manual of Mental Disorders* (Fourth Edition, Text Revision) (*DSM-IV-TR*)[1] can present differently across the lifespan. It has been demonstrated that young children are more likely to display hyperactive/impulsive symptoms versus inattention symptoms, and that the overall frequency of symptoms tends to decrease as a person gets older.[16,17]

Data suggest that there is an age-by-gender interaction in the presentation of ADHD symptoms. In other words, the presentation changes at different ages for boys versus girls. For example, the relative presentation of hyperactive/impulsive symptoms versus inattentive symptoms would be very different for a 7-year-old male compared to a 13-year-old female. As such, clinicians must rely on experience and clinical judgment to determine whether a given level of symptom presentation is developmentally inappropriate. Fortunately, clinicians can also use assessment instruments with normative data. These instruments allow clinicians to determine quantitatively how self, parent, or teacher reports of symptoms and related behaviors compare with age- and gender-matched normative information. This can be quite useful since often the threshold for determining developmental deviance is set to be 1.5–2 standard deviations from normative values for a particular age or gender group.

> Clinically, the take home message from the foregoing discussion is that due to the heterogeneous nature of ADHD, the presentation of symptoms can vary across ages and genders, and assessors must be mindful of these differences in order to make valid and reliable diagnoses.

Diagnostic process for the assessment of ADHD: *DSM-IV-TR*

Several different professional clinical organizations have published guidelines offering systematic descriptions of how to assess ADHD in children, adolescents, and adults.[18,19] Not surprisingly, these guidelines are largely organized around adherence to *DSM-IV-TR* diagnostic criteria. The following provides a summary of the five criteria (A–E) used within the *DSM-IV-TR* to classify ADHD, and the clinical approaches used to evaluate them.

Criterion A: Symptoms
A clinician must document the presence of at least six out of nine hyperactive–impulsive and/or at least six of nine inattentive symptoms (Table 1).[1] Assessing these symptoms is optimally done using both rating scales and clinical interviews. Rating scales, especially those with appropriate normative data, can bolster clinician judgment about developmental

deviance for a given patient. Best practice assessment, however, requires comprehensive follow-up interviews, and clinicians should never rely on rating scales alone to verify that this first criterion has been met. For children and adults, exhibiting overt hyperactivity, motor or verbal impulsivity, and/or attention problems during the clinic visit can often validate reports from the patient and others about the presence of symptoms. However, absence of such symptoms in the clinic does not necessarily mean the patient is asymptomatic. Even the most symptomatic and impaired patients can often "hold it together" in a novel setting to inhibit their ADHD symptoms. Therefore, it is important to obtain observation data about the patient's typical functioning in a variety of settings, including at home and at school or work. Rating scales offer a convenient way to obtain data from observers who are familiar with the patient's functioning in his or her usual settings. Clinician-administered structured and semi-structured interviews for assessing ADHD symptoms are also available for use with children, adolescents, and adults (see Chapter 3). These standardized interviews can support a thorough and appropriate evaluation of ADHD symptoms.

Table 1 Summary of *DSM-IV-TR* symptoms (Criterion A)

Inattention symptoms
• Often fails to give close attention to details or makes careless mistakes
• Often has difficulty sustaining attention
• Often does not seem to listen
• Often does not follow through on instructions, and fails to finish tasks
• Often has difficulty organizing activities
• Often avoids, dislikes, or is reluctant to engage in tasks requiring sustained attention
• Often loses things necessary for tasks or activities
• Is often easily distracted by extraneous stimuli
• Is often forgetful in daily activities
Hyperactivity/impulsivity symptoms
• Often fidgets with hands or feet
• Often leaves seats in situations where remaining seated is expected
• Often runs about or climbs excessively
• Often has difficulty engaging in leisure activities quietly
• Is often "on the go" or acts as if "driven by a motor"
• Often talks excessively
• Often blurts out answers before questions have been completed
• Often has difficulty waiting turn
• Often interrupts or intrudes on others

DSM-IV-TR, Diagnostic and Statistical Manual of Mental Disorders (Fourth Edition, Text Revision). Adapted from the American Psychiatric Association.[1]

Criterion B: Age of onset

The *DSM-IV-TR* criteria stipulate that there must be evidence of clinically impairing symptoms prior to the age of 7 years, although there is controversy over the validity of this criterion.[20-22] Clinically it is critical to establish chronicity of the disorder. Given the genetic and neurobiological underpinnings of ADHD, it is not a disorder that simply emerges in adolescence or adulthood, nor is its course intermittent. It is certainly possible that the clinical significance of symptoms may be less in childhood for some individuals. In any case, even for new cases that do not present until later in life, careful clinical interviewing is recommended to establish the presence of symptoms from early childhood as required for *DSM-IV-TR* diagnosis.

Criterion C: Pervasiveness

DSM-IV-TR requires that the symptoms are pervasive (ie, evident in at least two settings). ADHD is not a school-based disorder, nor is it confined to the workplace for adults. Careful assessment of pervasiveness can include the collection of data (often via rating scales) from multiple sources. For children and adolescents, these sources most typically include a parent and a teacher, but can also include coaches, youth leaders, close adult relatives, or other individuals who spend considerable time with the patient. In adults, it is important to collect patient self-report, as well as information from a significant other, co-worker, or close friend.

Criterion D: Clinically significant impairment

In order to meet the criteria for ADHD, the symptoms exhibited (and documented in Criterion A) must cause clear, clinically significant impairment in major role functions of the patient. For the child or adolescent, this typically refers to social, academic, and/or home functioning. In adolescents and adults, impairment can extend to occupational/vocational settings. For all ages, it is also possible for ADHD symptoms to cause impairment in the personal domain of functioning, wherein an individual's self-esteem or self-concept is markedly affected by their condition. The ability to easily discern clinically significant impairment may vary across clinical settings. For example, it may be easier to characterize impairment in a patient who is referred to a specialty provider than in a patient who complains of high levels of symptoms to a primary care provider. As with the other criteria, the best way to document clinically significant impairment is through interviewing the patient and other individuals in the patient's life (teachers, significant others, etc).

Criterion E: Ruling out additional disorders/differential diagnosis

It is critical to make sure that the symptoms observed in the patient are not better accounted for by other psychiatric/medical conditions. A number of the symptoms of ADHD are also present in a range of other psychiatric conditions, including depression, bipolar disorder, anxiety disorders, and substance abuse disorders. Moreover, the impairments caused by ADHD are often similar to those manifested in these other conditions. Careful diagnostic interviewing with structured or semi-structured interviews is an efficient way to assess for other psychiatric conditions. In addition, gathering a comprehensive medical history can help determine whether additional physical exams or other testing may be necessary to rule out medical problems that could account for observed symptoms.

2 Rating scales for the assessment of ADHD

Why use rating scales for the diagnostic assessment of ADHD?

Rating scales can be a valuable tool for making a valid diagnosis of ADHD in children, adolescents, and adults. Specifically, rating scales can provide information pertaining to two of the aforementioned *DSM-IV-TR* criteria for ADHD criteria A and C. For Criterion A, scales with normative data can be used to determine whether a patient is exhibiting symptoms that are statistically more deviant than their age- and gender-matched peers. Criterion C can be evaluated by having raters from different domains of a patient's life (eg, parents or teachers for children; co-workers or spouses for adults) complete the forms to describe the pervasiveness of the symptoms. These clinical data, when supplemented with appropriate follow-up clinical interviewing, can be an efficient way to collect meaningful information to make diagnostic decisions.

Using assessment scales to monitor treatment response

In addition to using rating scales to establish initial diagnosis of ADHD, they can also be useful instruments to monitor ongoing treatment response by assessing changes in symptom ratings. Results from any rating scale can be compared qualitatively over time to evaluate whether a treatment is showing effect for a given patient. It is possible, for example, for a person's ADHD impairment to be driven largely by only a few symptoms; if treatment results in broad-based symptom reduction but does not address these specific problems, the clinician may need to revise the treatment plan. Also, since some scales measure the impairments or impact of ADHD on quality of life, they can be used as a complement to symptom-based rating scales to monitor treatment progress.

Selecting a rating scale

There are several important considerations when selecting a rating scale, including scale features and supporting documentation. Features of the rating scales include the purpose of the scale, age range for patients, and rater types. Age range varies by rating scale, as do rater types. Supporting documentation is important, as it helps establish a level of confidence in results obtained with a rating scale. Examples of supporting documentation include peer-reviewed publications and manuals that describe the standardization process for the rating scale and normative data.

Availability of a relevant normative sample is also an important consideration in supporting documentation. When a normative sample (or "norms") describes a representative sample of people (eg, by age, gender, or race/ethnicity), a patient's results can be compared with the norms to help establish whether the patient has unusual levels of ADHD symptoms. It is also helpful to know how the scale performs for people with other disorders, particularly disorders that might be considered in differential diagnosis.

Rating scales for children and adolescents

A number of scales have been developed to assess the signs and symptoms of ADHD in children and adolescents. Some of these are focused on ADHD and related issues; others include ADHD among a broader spectrum of concerns (Table 2).

Conners 3rd edition

The Conners 3rd edition (Conners 3)[31] is the updated version of the well-known Conners Rating Scales – Revised (CRS-R).[31] Various versions of the Conners rating scales have been used in ADHD assessments since the 1960s, and this most recent edition was published in 2008. This focused ADHD assessment tool includes *DSM-IV-TR* symptoms of ADHD as well as oppositional defiant disorder (ODD) and conduct disorder (CD). The Conners 3 also includes related issues, such as executive functioning and social problems. This rating scale is appropriate for rating school-aged youth who are 6–18 years old, and can be completed by patients, parents, and teachers. It is available in English and Spanish, with some forms available in French.

Structure and format
Elements of the Conners 3 include the following:
- four *DSM-IV-TR* scales (ADHD inattentive, ADHD hyperactive/impulsive, CD, and ODD) that include items corresponding to each *DSM-IV-TR* symptom for these disorders;
- content scales representing key constructs in ADHD (inattention, hyperactivity/impulsivity, learning problems, executive functioning, defiance/aggression, peer relations [parent and teacher forms], and family relations [self-report form]);
- two index scales, the Conners 3 ADHD index (Conners 3AI; how similar a child is to the clinical ADHD sample) and the Conners 3 global index (Conners 3GI; assessment of global functioning, same items as used historically on the Conners scales), which has two subscales (restless–impulsive, emotional lability);
- three validity scales (positive impression, negative impression, and inconsistency index) to capture potential rater bias or extreme response styles;
- severe conduct critical items;

Table 2 Summary of rating scales used to assess ADHD and related impairments in children and adolescents

Scale name	Source	Age range	Administration: modalities, time required, and number of items	Parent	Teacher	Self-report	DSM	Normative data and psychometric properties	Notes
				Rater types					
Achenbach System of Empirically Based Assessment (ASEBA)	Commercially available	1.5 to 90 years and older	Online, software, paper–pencil 10–90 mins 99–112 problem items	✓	✓	✓	*	Age- and gender-based norms; primarily empirically derived factors; demonstrated reliability and validity; good discriminative validity	Reading level is 5th grade Online, software, and hand-scoring are available
ADD-H Comprehensive Teacher's Rating Scale, 2nd Edition (ACTeRS)	Commercially available	Grades K-adult	Paper–pencil 10–15 mins 24–35 items	✓	✓	✓	X	Limited normative sample; empirically derived factor structure; limited information regarding reliability and validity; further study needed	Reading level is not reported No normative data for use of the self-report with adolescents Hand-scored
ADHD Rating Scale-IV (ADHD-RS-IV)	Commercially available	5–18 years	Paper–pencil 10 mins 18 items	✓	✓	X	✓	Has age- and gender-based norms; based on DSM-IV (not empirically derived factor structure); demonstrated reliability and validity; demonstrated specificity and sensitivity for identifying potential ADHD	Reading level is not reported Preschool version (3–5 years old) described in research; not commercially available at this time Hand-scored

Scale	Availability	Age range	Format					Psychometric properties	Comments
ADHD Symptom Checklist-4 (ADHD-SC4)	Commercially available	3–18 years	Paper–pencil 10–15 mins 50 items	✓	✓		X	Normative data limited; based on DSM-IV (not empirically derived factor structure); variable reliability and validity; data require further study; good sensitivity but poor specificity for identifying potential ADHD	Reading level is not reported; No normative data reported for teacher ratings of 13 to 18 year olds; geographically limited normative samples; Hand-scored
Behavior Assessment System for Children, Second edition (BASC-2)	Commercially available	2–21 years (6 years– college for self-report)	Paper–pencil 10–30 mins 100–176 items	✓	✓	✓	X	Age- and gender-based norms available; authors recommend use of combined gender norms; empirically derived factors; demonstrated reliability and validity; scales do not consistently discriminate among expected clinical groups	Reading level is 2nd grade (child and adolescent self-report), 4th grade (P); other forms not reported; Software and hand-scoring available
Brown Attention-Deficit Disorder Scales for Children and Adolescents (Brown ADD Scales)	Commercially available	3–18 years	Paper–pencil, online 10–20 mins 40–50 items	✓ †	✓ †	✓	X	Limited normative data; empirically derived factor structure; demonstrated reliability and validity; good specificity but poor sensitivity for identifying potential ADHD in adolescents; discriminative data not available for younger children	Reading level is not reported; Downward extension of the Brown Attention Deficit Disorder Scales for Adolescents and Adults; Software and hand-scoring available

(Continues overleaf).

Table 2 Summary of rating scales used to assess ADHD and related impairments in children and adolescents (continued)

Scale name	Source	Age range	Administration: modalities, time required, and number of items	Parent	Teacher	Self-report	DSM	Normative data and psychometric properties	Notes
					Rater types				
Conners 3rd Edition (Conners 3)	Commercially available	6–18 years (8–18 years for self-report)	Online, paper–pencil 5–25 mins *Conners 3 (full-length)*: 99–115 items *Conners 3(S)*: 41–45 items *Conners 3AI*: 10 items *Conners 3GI*: 10 items (P & T)	✓	✓	✓	✓	Has age- and gender-based norms; some empirically derived factors, some *DSM*-based factors; demonstrated reliability and validity; demonstrated specificity and sensitivity for identifying potential ADHD	Reading level is 3rd grade (self-report), 4th–5th grade (P & T) Online, software, and hand-scoring available
Conners Comprehensive Behavior Rating Scales (Conners CBRS)	Commercially available	6–18 years (8–18 self-report)	Online, paper–pencil 10–25 mins *Conners CBRS*: 179–204 items *Conners CI*: 24 items	✓	✓	✓	✓	Age- and gender-based norms; some empirically derived factors; some *DSM*-based factors; demonstrated reliability and validity; demonstrated specificity and sensitivity for identifying potential disorders, including ADHD	Reading level is 3rd grade (self-report), 4th grade (P & T) Online, software, and hand-scoring available

Scale	Availability	Age	Administration					Normative/psychometric data	Notes
Conners Early Childhood (Conners EC)	Commercially available	2–6 years	Online, paper–pencil 5–25 mins *Conners EC (full-length):* 186–190 items *Conners EC BEH:* 115–116 items *Conners EC BEH(S):* 48–49 items *Conners EC DM:* 74–80 items *Conners ECGI:* 10 items	✓	✓	✗	✓	Age- and gender-based norms; empirically derived factor structure; demonstrated reliability and validity; demonstrated specificity and sensitivity for identifying potential disorders, including ADHD	Reading level is 5th grade Online, software, and hand-scoring available
Swanson, Nolan, & Pelham-IV Teacher and Parent Rating Scale (SNAP-IV)	Available from author's website	6–12 years	Paper–pencil 15 mins 10–90 items	✓	✓	✗	✓	Limited normative data; some empirically derived factors, some *DSM*-based factors; limited psychometric data available for review – further study needed	Reading level is 3rd grade (P); not reported for teacher form No manual available Some sources report 6–18 years age range, but normative data and psychometric data are not reported for children over 12 years of age Hand-scored
Vanderbilt ADHD Diagnostic Parent/Teacher Rating Scales (VADPRS, VADTRS)	Commercially available through AAP bookstore	6–12 years	Paper–pencil 10 mins 43–55 items	✓	✓	✗	✓	No normative data; based on *DSM-IV* (not empirically derived factor structure); further study of psychometrics needed	Reading level is below 3rd grade (P), not reported for teacher form No manual available Hand-scored

(Continued). *"*DSM*-oriented" scales include items rated by at least 14 out of 22 psychiatrists as being "very consistent" with *DSM-IV* criteria; † Adolescent version is self-report only; no form or normative data available for P or T ratings of this age group. AAP, American Academy of Pediatrics; AI, ADHD index; ADD-H, attention deficit disorder-hyperactivity; BEH, behavior scales; BEH(S), short behavior scales; CI, clinical index; DM, developmental milestones; ECGI, early childhood global index; GI, global index; K, kindergarten; P, parent form; T, teacher form; S, short form. Adapted from Achenbach et al;[23] Achenbach et al;[24] Ullmann et al;[25] DuPaul et al;[26] Gadow et al;[27] Reynolds et al;[28] Brown;[29] Brown;[30] Conners;[31] Conners;[32] Conners;[33] Swanson et al;[34] Wolraich et al;[35] and Wolraich et al.[36]

- screener items for anxiety and for depression;
- three impairment items (home, school, social); and
- two additional questions (other concerns, strengths, and skills).

The full-length Conners 3 includes all of these elements and has about 100 items. There is a short form of the Conners 3 – Conners 3(S) – that has abbreviated versions of the content scales, as well as two validity scales and the two additional questions. The Conners 3AI form can be rated by parents, teachers, and patients, and is 10 items long. The Conners 3GI form is also 10 items long, and can be rated by parents and teachers. Each item on the Conners 3 is rated on a scale of 0 to 3, with 3 indicating very high frequency/severity.

Scoring and interpretation

The computerized scoring options produce reports of results, including suggested interpretation guidelines. The progress report includes the reliable change index, which statistically compares more than one administration of the Conners 3; this is useful when assessing response to treatment. The comparative report notes statistically significant differences among raters describing the same child.

Normative data are available for the Conners 3, separated by age (1-year groups) and gender; a combined gender option is available. Raw scores can be compared with the norms to calculate *T*-scores and percentiles as a way to establish whether symptoms are typical or atypical for that child's age/gender. A high score on any Conners 3 scale indicates high levels of concern in that area. There is no single summary score for the total Conners 3; each scale produces a separate score.

Pros, cons, and best uses

The Conners 3 is supported by a long history of research, solid psychometrics, reasonable normative samples, and a comprehensive manual. The use of small age bands (1 year) in normative data provides greater accuracy in describing a child's functioning relative to peers. Overall correct classification rates for the Conners 3AI are 83% (parent), 79% (teacher), and 77% (self-report).[37] Three validity scales on the Conners 3 help identify extreme response bias on the rater's part.

Because the Conners 3 was recently released, no data have been published regarding sensitivity to treatment. The 10 items on the Conners 3GI are identical to those on the CRS-R Conners GI, suggesting that this index should continue to be sensitive to treatment for ADHD.[31] Although the full-length Conners 3 is long for repeated administration, there are shorter forms available for this purpose.

The Conners 3 is recommended for use when assessing for possible ADHD. The full-length form offers relevant *DSM-IV-TR* symptoms of ADHD, ODD, and CD, which informs of possible comorbidity with the disruptive behavior disorders. Content scales provide guidance as to accompanying issues that may need attention in the treatment plan.

Useful resource
Further information about the Conners 3 can be found at www.mhs.com.

Conners Comprehensive Behavior Rating Scales

The Conners Comprehensive Behavior Rating Scales (Conners CBRS)[32] were developed simultaneously with the Conners 3 (see above). The Conners CBRS is a broadband assessment tool that includes *DSM-IV-TR* symptoms of ADHD along with symptoms of many other *DSM-IV-TR* diagnoses. There is a physical symptoms scale that includes common side effects of psychoactive medications. Relevant associated issues of ADHD are also covered, though not in the same depth as on the Conners 3. Like the Conners 3, this rating scale is appropriate for rating school-aged youth who are 6–18 years old, and can be completed by patients, parents, and teachers. It is available in English and Spanish, with some forms available in French.

Structure and format
Elements of the Conners CBRS include the following:
- 12 *DSM-IV-TR* scales (ADHD inattentive, ADHD hyperactive/impulsive, CD, ODD, major depressive episode, manic episode, generalized anxiety disorder, separation anxiety disorder, social phobia, obsessive–compulsive disorder, autistic disorder, and Asperger's disorder) that include items corresponding to each *DSM-IV-TR* symptom for these disorders/episodes;
- content scales representing key clinical constructs (hyperactivity/impulsivity, academic difficulties, defiant/aggressive behaviors, emotional distress, social problems, perfectionistic and compulsive behaviors, physical symptoms, and violence potential indicator);
- one index scale, the Conners clinical index (Conners CI), that describes how similar a child is to the clinical samples versus the general population sample;
- three validity scales (positive impression, negative impression, and inconsistency index) intended to capture potential rater bias or extreme response styles;
- severe conduct critical items;
- self-harm critical items;
- other clinical indicators representing issues like bullying, pica, and tics;
- three impairment items (home, school, social); and
- two additional questions (other concerns, and strengths and skills).

The full-length Conners CBRS includes all of these elements and has about 200 items. The Conners CI form is just 24 items long. Each form can be rated by parents, teachers, and patients. Each item on the Conners CBRS is rated on a scale of 0 to 3, with 3 indicating very high frequency/severity.

Scoring and interpretation
The computerized scoring options produce reports of results, including suggested interpretation guidelines. The progress report includes the reliable change index, which

statistically compares more than one administration of the Conners CBRS; this is useful when assessing response to treatment. The comparative report notes statistically significant differences among raters describing the same child.

Normative data are available for the Conners CBRS, separated by age (1-year groups) and gender; a combined gender option is available. Raw scores can be compared with the norms to calculate T-scores and percentiles as a way to establish whether symptoms are typical or atypical for that child's age/gender. A high score on any Conners CBRS scale indicates high levels of concern in that area. There is no single summary score for the total Conners CBRS; each scale produces a separate score.

Pros, cons, and best uses

The Conners CBRS is supported by solid psychometrics, reasonable normative samples, and a comprehensive manual. The use of small age bands (1 year) in normative data provides greater accuracy in describing a child's functioning relative to peers. Overall correct classification rates for the five Conners CI Indicators are good (in order of parent, teacher, and self-report forms: disruptive behavior disorder indicator 83%, 79%, 77%; learning and language disorder indicator 85%, 82%, 83%; mood disorder indicator 89%, 85%, 77%; anxiety disorder indicator 70%, 76%, 82%; and ADHD indicator 84%, 74%, 78%).[37] Three validity scales on the Conners CBRS help identify extreme response bias on the rater's part. The Conners CBRS is convenient to score and interpret, as it is readily available through a number of suppliers.

Because the Conners CBRS was recently released, no data have been published regarding sensitivity to treatment. The length of the Conners CBRS is also prohibitive for frequent use in treatment monitoring; however, it is a valuable asset when conducting a broad survey of important issues for children in the 6–18 year age range.

The Conners CBRS is recommended for use when surveying a number of diagnostic possibilities, including ADHD, as most of the key differential diagnosis considerations are represented with the exception of childhood psychosis.

Useful resource
The Conners CBRS can be found at www.mhs.com.

Conners Early Childhood

The Conners Early Childhood scale (Conners EC)[33] is a broadband assessment tool for behavioral, emotional, social, cognitive, and developmental issues that arise in early childhood. It is not diagnosis-specific, although it does include constructs relevant to ADHD like inattention and hyperactivity. It also has a physical symptoms scale that includes common side effects of psychoactive medications. The Conners EC can be completed by parents, teachers, and childcare providers to describe young children who are 2–6 years old. It is available in English and Spanish, with some forms available in French.

Structure and format

Elements of the Conners EC include the following:

- six behavior scales (inattention/hyperactivity, defiant/aggressive behaviors, social functioning/atypical behaviors, anxiety, mood and affect, and physical symptoms);
- five developmental milestone scales (adaptive skills, communication, motor skills, play, and pre-academic/cognitive);
- one index scale, the Conners ECGI (assessment of global functioning, same items as used historically on the Conners scales), which has two subscales (restless-impulsive and emotional lability);
- three validity scales (positive impression, negative impression, and inconsistency index) intended to capture potential rater bias or extreme response styles;
- other clinical indicators representing issues like cruelty to animals, pica, and self-injury;
- three impairment items (home, learning/pre-academic, peer interactions); and
- two additional questions (other concerns, and strengths and skills).

The full-length Conners EC includes all of these elements and has about 190 items. There is a Conners Behavior scales form (Conners EC BEH) that omits the developmental milestone scales. The Conners BEH(S) form is a short version of the Conners EC BEH form that includes abbreviated versions of the behavior scales as well as two of the validity scales and the two additional questions, for a total of 49 items. The Conners EC developmental milestones form (Conners EC DM) has the developmental milestone scales, impairment items, and additional questions. The Conners ECGI is 10 items long, and can be rated by parents and teachers.

There are parent and childcare provider/teacher forms for each version of the Conners EC. Most items on the Conners EC are rated on a scale of 0 to 3, with 3 indicating very high frequency/severity. The developmental milestone items are rated on a scale of 0 to 2, with 0 indicating no demonstration of a skill, 1 indicating inconsistent demonstration or the need for help, and 2 indicating consistent and independent demonstration of the skill.

Scoring and interpretation

The computerized scoring options produce reports of results, including suggested interpretation guidelines. The progress report includes the reliable change index, which statistically compares more than one administration of the Conners EC; this is useful when assessing response to treatment. The comparative report notes statistically significant differences among raters describing the same child.

Normative data are available for the Conners EC, separated by age (6-month groups) and gender; a combined gender option is available. Raw scores can be compared with the norms to calculate *T*-scores and percentiles as a way to establish whether symptoms are typical or atypical for that child's age/gender. A high score on any Conners EC scale indicates high levels of concern in that area. There is no single summary score for the total Conners EC; each scale produces a separate score.

Pros, cons, and best uses

The Conners EC has solid psychometrics, reasonable normative samples, and a comprehensive manual. The use of small age bands (6 months) in normative data provides accuracy in describing a child's functioning relative to peers. The mean overall correct classification rate for the Conners EC, averaged across all scales and across all rater types, is 86%.[37] Three validity scales on the Conners EC help identify extreme response bias on the rater's part. The Conners EC is convenient to score and interpret, and it is readily available through a number of suppliers.

Because the Conners EC was recently released, no data have been published regarding sensitivity to treatment. The 10 items on the Conners ECGI are identical to those on the CRS-R Conners GI, suggesting that this index should continue to be sensitive to treatment for ADHD.[33]

The Conners EC is recommended for use when collecting data about a number of domains of functioning for young children, including ways that ADHD may be manifested in early childhood.

Useful resource

The Conners EC can be found at www.mhs.com.

Vanderbilt ADHD Diagnostic Parent/Teacher Rating Scales

The Vanderbilt ADHD Diagnostic Parent Rating Scale (VADPRS)[35] and Teacher Rating Scale (VADTRS)[36] are focused rating scales for the assessment of *DSM-IV*[38] symptoms of ADHD. Symptoms of ODD, CD, anxiety, and depression are also included. This rating scale was designed for use with children ages 6–12 years old, and has forms for parent- and teacher-ratings. It is available in English and Spanish.

Structure and format

Items on the VADPRS/VADTRS are presented to raters in the following groups:

- predominantly inattentive subtype;
- predominantly hyperactive/impulsive subtype;
- combined subtype;
- ODD and CD (separate clusters on the VADPRS);
- anxiety or depression; and
- a "performance" section that is used to assess impairment.

The parent form has 47 items rated from 0 to 3 (3 indicating "very often"), plus 3 academic performance items and 5 classroom behavior items rated from 0 to 5 (5 indicating above average behavior/performance). The teacher form has 35 items rated from 0 to 3, with 3 academic performance items and 5 classroom behavior items rated from 0 to 5 (5 indicating above average behavior/performance).

Scoring and interpretation

Scoring instructions are provided with each hardcopy form, specifying how many items must be "counted behaviors" (ie, rated a 2 or 3) in each cluster before a diagnosis can be considered.

Normative data are not available in a manual format, but some samples have been described in the research literature.[35,36]

Raw scores are not summed on VADPRS and VADTRS; rather, a recommended cut-off is provided; for example, "Requires 6 or more counted behaviors from questions 1 through 9 for indication of...". High scores on most of the items indicate high frequency of undesired behaviors; high scores on the 8 performance items indicate good performance.

Pros, cons, and best uses

The VADPRS and VADTRS are brief, focused rating scales for ADHD symptoms. They are recommended for use primarily in research settings and in screening large numbers of children. Until further data are published, caution is urged in using these scales for clinical assessment and individual treatment monitoring.

There are no manuals for the VADPRS or VADTRS, but each form has a single sheet with scoring instructions. There is no standardized administration procedure, and various versions of the rating scales vary in their instructions (eg, some specify "in the past 6 months," some "in the past month," and others do not specify a time frame). Normative data are not currently available for comparison with individual patient results. Preliminary data suggest reasonable internal consistency and convergent validity, but further study needs to be done to determine psychometric properties. Treatment sensitivity is unknown.

> **Useful resource**
> VADPRS and VADTRS forms can be ordered through the American Academy of Pediatrics bookstore (www.aap.org/bookstorepubs.html; search "NICHQ Vanderbilt Assessment Scale").

ADHD Rating Scale-IV

The ADHD Rating Scale-IV (ADHD-RS-IV)[26] focuses on the 18 symptoms of ADHD from the *DSM-IV-TR*. It was developed as a rating scale for completion by parents and teachers about children who are 5–18 years old. The ADHD-RS-IV home version is available in English or Spanish; the school version is available in English. A modification of the ADHD-RS-IV for use with adults is discussed on page 29. Some research projects use an investigator-completed version of the ADHD-RS-IV.[39,40]

Structure and format

The ADHD-RS-IV has items representing two *DSM-IV* subtypes of ADHD:
- inattention (9 *DSM* symptoms); and
- hyperactivity/impulsivity (9 *DSM* symptoms).

This rating scale has 18 items, with one item for each *DSM-IV-TR* symptom of ADHD. The standard form presents these 18 items in alternating order (ie, odd-numbered items represent inattention symptoms, even-numbered items the hyperactivity/impulsivity symptoms). Note that other versions have been prepared for various research studies, and thus the order of items may have been changed. Each item is rated on a 4-point frequency scale ranging from 0 ("never or rarely") to 3 ("very often").

Scoring and interpretation

Standard clinical administration includes instructions to rate the items based on the child's behavior in the past 6 months or "since the beginning of the school year" if the teacher has known the child less than 6 months. This time frame is sometimes changed for research or treatment-monitoring purposes, but this prevents use of the normative data.

Three scales are available: total, inattention, and hyperactivity/impulsivity. The ratings for items on each scale are summed, then this raw score is compared to the appropriate scoring table for normative data (based on ≥3-year age bands and gender) and converted to percentiles. When a raw score is associated with more than one percentile, the lowest percentile should be reported. The test manual and research publications by the scale developers recommend using different cut-off scores for different contexts (eg, clinical work versus research studies).[41] Research on the ADHD-RS-IV suggests that both parent and teacher ratings should be used in identifying children with ADHD.[41] A high score on the ADHD-RS-IV indicates high frequency of ADHD symptoms.

Pros, cons, and best uses

The ADHD-RS-IV has a readily available manual and published manuscripts describing reasonable psychometrics and normative sample supporting its use as a parent and teacher rating scale.[26,42–44] Data from a small clinical sample suggest reasonable treatment sensitivity for the ADHD-RS-IV, with an indication that parent ratings may be more sensitive than teacher ratings in this particular study.[45]

On the standard form, alternation of items from the two symptom sets may help reduce response bias regarding ADHD subtypes, but is unlikely to reduce bias from the perspective of "ADHD or not." Many non-standard forms are in circulation (including so-called "clinician-rated" or "investigator" versions); caution should be used when interpreting results from these forms as they do not correspond with published normative data and psychometric studies.

The ADHD-RS-IV is easily used as a rating scale for completion by parents and teachers, with straight-forward scoring and interpretation. It is a useful way to quickly gather data on the 18 symptoms of ADHD from the *DSM-IV-TR*, with a large normative sample to help establish whether symptoms are developmentally inappropriate. The reliable change index calculation discussed in the manual is a useful way to quantify change after intervention.

Indications are that the parent- and teacher-rated ADHD-RS-IV may be sensitive to treatment-related change; if further data with larger samples support these findings, this rating scale will be a useful tool for treatment monitoring. Be cautious when reviewing research publications that mention use of the ADHD-RS-IV, as many pharmaceutical studies employ an investigator-rated version based on interview and/or observation data, and findings with that variation are not applicable to parent- and teacher-rated forms.

Useful resource

The ADHD-RS-IV manual can be ordered from the publisher at www.guilford.com.

Swanson, Nolan, & Pelham-IV Teacher and Parent Rating Scale

The Swanson, Nolan, & Pelham-IV Teacher and Parent Rating Scale (SNAP-IV)[34] focuses on ADHD and ODD symptoms from the *DSM-IV*, with additional items to aid with differential diagnostic decisions. The SNAP-IV is intended for use with children (reported age range varies from 6–12 years old to 6–18 years old), and can be completed by parents and teachers. It was developed in English, and has been translated into Spanish, German, French, Chinese, and Italian. The SNAP[46] was originally developed to correspond with *Diagnostic and Statistical Manual of Mental Disorders* (Third Edition)[47] criteria,[46] and updated to reflect *Diagnostic and Statistical Manual of Mental Disorders* (Third Edition Revised)[48] and then *DSM-IV*[88] criteria.

Structure and format

Items on the SNAP-IV are presented to raters in the following groups:
- ADHD inattention;
- ADHD hyperactivity/impulsivity;
- ODD; and
- screening items for possible differential diagnoses, including CD, anxiety disorders, and mood disorders.

Based on analyses of other data sets, 10 items adapted from a previous version of the Conners rating scales (IOWA Conners or CLAM [Conners, Loney, and Milich])[49] can be scored to obtain the inattention/overactivity index (I/O) and aggression/defiance index (A/D). In addition, a "Conners Index" can be calculated using 10 items from the SNAP-IV (note that the so-called "Conners Index" on the SNAP-IV contains different items than those on the Conners 3 and Conners EC indices).

The complete SNAP-IV is 90 items long. A short 26-item form (ie, "MTA version" or "SNAP-IV-26") has also been used, including items from the ADHD and ODD scales. A short form – known as the Swanson, Kotkin, Agler, M-Flynn and Pelham Scale (SKAMP)[50] – is also available based on 10 items of the SNAP-IV. The SKAMP is intended to estimate the severity of ADHD symptoms in the classroom.[50] SNAP-IV forms for parents versus teachers do not differ. Each item on the SNAP-IV is rated on a 4-point scale ranging from "not at all" to "very much." Most of the items include frequency terms (eg, "often," "sometimes").

Scoring and interpretation

Each SNAP-IV item rating is converted to a raw score of 0 to 3, 0 being "not at all," and written on the hand-scoring template. These raw item scores are added to obtain the total raw scores for each of the scales described above. The two ADHD scales are added to obtain an ADHD combined raw score. An average rating-per-item is calculated for each of these scales.

The scoring instructions include "tentative 5% cut-offs" for the average rating on each *DSM-IV*-based scale; however, the basis for these cut-off scores is reportedly a sample of low income Hispanic elementary school students.[51] The authors suggest alternative revised cut-off scores based on a research sample; those scores are described in Table 3.[51] A high score on the SNAP-IV scales indicates high frequency of the behaviors. There is no single summary score for the total SNAP-IV; each scale produces a separate score.

Pros, cons, and best uses

There is no manual available for the SNAP-IV; however, online scoring instructions are available. Although the SNAP-IV is reportedly for use with 6- to 18-year-old patients, normative sample and limited psychometrics are reported for elementary school children only. Preliminary data suggest scores may vary by gender, race, and socioeconomic status.[51] Using the 5% cut-off may result in over-identification of cases.[52] Published data suggest that the SNAP-IV is sensitive to medication-related change.[53–55]

In short, the SNAP-IV may be appropriate for screening large numbers of students to identify those who may require individual assessment. It also appears useful for assessing change in research studies. Until additional normative and psychometric data are available, caution is urged in using the SNAP-IV for clinical assessment and individual treatment monitoring.

Useful resource

The SNAP-IV forms and instructions can be found at www.ADHD.net.

Table 3 The suggested revised cut-off scores for SNAP-IV

	ADHD-inattention (average rating)	ADHD-hyperactivity/ impulsivity (average rating)	Recommendation
Parent or teacher	>1.2	>1.2	If either cut-off is exceeded for either rater type, recommend diagnostic assessment for ADHD
Parent data only	>2.4	>1.8	If either cut-off is exceeded for parent ratings, increased probability of an ADHD diagnosis

Adapted from Bussing et al.[51]

ADHD Symptom Checklist-4

The ADHD Symptom Checklist-4 (ADHD-SC4)[27] is a focused assessment tool for ADHD, including items reflecting *DSM-IV* symptoms of ADHD and ODD. The ADHD-SC4 is part of a series of child symptom inventories. Some of the items on the checklist are reworded to be shorter than the original versions on the child symptom inventories. The ADHD-SC4 is used to describe symptoms in children aged 3–18 years old. Parents and teachers complete the same form, which is available in English and Spanish.

Structure and format

The ADHD-SC4 response form presents 50 items divided into the following groups:
- *DSM-IV* ADHD (18 items: 1–9 inattention, items 10–18 hyperactivity/impulsivity);
- *DSM-IV* ODD (8 items);
- peer conflict (10 items, including some symptoms of CD); and
- stimulant side effects checklist (14 items, including mood, behavioral, and physical symptoms).

Three index scores can be obtained: mood, attention–arousal, and physical complaints. Each item is rated on a 4-point scale ranging from "never" to "very often."

Scoring and interpretation

There are two ways to score results from the ADHD-SC4: "screening cut-off" (ie, "symptom count" score) and "symptom severity" score. The screening cut-off approach involves converting each item response to a "0" (absent) or "1" (present). These are used to count the number of symptoms present for each category; this symptom count is compared with a *DSM*-based "symptom criterion score" to determine if further evaluation is recommended.

In contrast, the symptom severity score is obtained when item ratings are converted into item raw scores, which are added for each category, then converted into *T*-scores and percentiles. Separate scores are obtained for ADHD inattentive type, ADHD hyperactive type, ADHD combined type, ODD, and peer conflict. *T*-scores and raw scores can be summarized on "Symptom Severity Profile" score sheets. For either scoring approach, a high score indicates higher frequency/severity of symptoms.

Pros, cons, and best uses

The ADHD-SC4 manual[27] provides background on the scales, psychometric data, normative data, scoring information, and clinical applications. Normative data are available to compare a child's results with the general population or with a clinical sample (including ADHD and ODD). A study by the test's authors reported good sensitivity but poor specificity for ADHD when screening cut-off scores were used (ie, correctly identified 91% of the ADHD cases, but incorrectly labeled 64% of the general population as ADHD),[56] indicating that these cut-off scores may overidentify ADHD in the general population. A published study showed the ADHD-SC4 was sensitive to medication-related change in hyperactivity.[57]

Of concern, the term "ADHD" is included in the header of each form, which could contribute to response bias. Also, items are grouped by diagnosis, which can lead to response set, although a study by the test authors found no significant differences in results when test items were administered in a randomized order versus structured by construct.[58]

Overall, the ADHD-SC4 is a relatively brief, well-established checklist that includes *DSM-IV* symptoms of ADHD. The stimulant side effects checklist makes this tool particularly helpful when a treatment plan includes a stimulant medication. This scale may be a useful way to monitor symptoms over time or change in response to treatment, as well as serving as a quick screen for possible ADHD. If using this measure for screening, remember the high rate of false positives associated with the screening cut-off scores identified in the manual.

Useful resource

The forms and manual for the ADHD-SC4 are available at www.checkmateplus.com.

Attention Deficit Disorder with Hyperactivity Comprehensive Teacher Rating Scale

The Attention Deficit Disorder with Hyperactivity Comprehensive Teacher Rating Scale (ACTeRS)[25] is a focused rating scale for features of ADHD (including inattention and hyperactivity) and related issues (including social skills, oppositional behavior, and early childhood behavior). Although the original version was created for teacher ratings in the classroom, the current version includes parent, teacher, and self-report forms. Parent and teacher forms are available in English and Spanish, and can be used to describe youth who are kindergarten through 8th grade (5–14 years old). There is also a self-report form that can be completed by adolescents (≥12 years old) and adults.

Structure and format

Items on parent (25 items) and teacher (24 items) forms of the ACTeRS are presented to the rater in the following sections:

- attention;
- hyperactivity;
- social skills; and
- oppositional behavior.

The parent form also has an early childhood behavior section. The self-report form has 35 items that are scored on three scales: attention, hyperactivity/impulsivity, and social adjustment. Each item is rated on a 5-point frequency scale, ranging from "almost never" (1) to "almost always" (5).

Scoring and interpretation

Raw item scores are summed for each scale and converted into percentiles or *T*-scores using normative data. The manual recommends assigning a diagnosis of "ADD" when the attention subscale is at or below the 10th percentile.

Parent and teacher norms are separated by gender; self-report norms are not separated by gender. A low percentile score on the ACTeRS indicates greater severity of problems.

Pros, cons, and best uses

Overall, despite some attractive features, clinical use of the ACTeRS is limited by several factors. These include limited information about normative sample and clinical samples, lack of complete normative sample, and limited data regarding test–retest reliability (parent form), discriminative validity, and treatment sensitivity. Each scale on the ACTeRS has very few items (4 to 7 items per scale on the parent and teacher forms), which limits interpretation of the scores. Furthermore, the ACTeRS is not clearly linked to *DSM-IV-TR* constructs, which limits its use for diagnostic assessment.

Useful resource

The most recent edition of the ACTeRS is available from the publisher at www.metritech.com.

Brown Attention Deficit Disorder Scales

The Brown Attention Deficit Disorder Scales (Brown ADD Scales)[29,30] model ADD as a complex disorder of executive functioning rather than on the *DSM-IV-TR* view of ADHD. The scales can be administered as rating scales or as clinical interviews, and are available for four age ranges: primary/preschool (ages 3–7), school-age (ages 8–12), adolescent (ages 12–18), and adult (≥18; please see page 32 for the use of the Brown ADD Scales for adult patients). The primary/preschool and school-age versions can be rated by parents and teachers, with a self-report form available for children aged 8–12 years. The adolescent and adult forms are self-rated, or can be completed by a "collateral" source. A "Brown ADD Diagnostic Form" is also available to guide data collection for a comprehensive evaluation, including clinical history, comorbidity screener, and worksheet for combining Brown ADD Scales data with other test data.

Structure and format

All forms of the Brown ADD Scales include five clusters of executive functioning:
- organizing, prioritizing, and activating to work;
- focusing, sustaining, and shifting attention to tasks;
- regulating alertness, sustaining effort, and processing speed;
- managing frustration and modulating emotions; and
- utilizing working memory and accessing recall.

The primary/preschool and school-age forms add a 6th cluster: monitoring and self-regulating action. Each Brown ADD Scales form is 40–50 items long (primary/preschool 44 items, school-age 50 items, adolescent 40 items, and adult 40 items). Each item is rated on a 4-point scale describing frequency in the past week (0, never; 1, once a week or less; 2, twice a week; 3, almost daily).

Scoring and interpretation

The raw item scores in each cluster are summed, then converted to a *T*-score for each cluster. The raw sums from the five main clusters are added together and converted to a *T*-score for the "ADD-inattention total score." For the two childhood versions, the sum of all items is converted to a *T*-score labeled the "ADD-combined total score." This *T*-score can be categorized using guidelines in the manual (with *T* ≥55 indicating "ADD highly probable"). The computerized scoring option also provides a report of results, including graphs. In addition, the computer software allows comparison of multiple reports from different raters or from different points in time. A high score on the Brown ADD Scales indicates higher levels of impairment in these domains.

Pros, cons, and best uses

Manuals are available for the various versions of the Brown ADD Scales, each describing the normative sample(s), clinical samples, and psychometric data. Caution should be used when applying recommended cut-off scores from the manual, as these may underidentify cases of ADHD; for example, in one study nearly 50% of subjects who were diagnosed with ADHD-inattentive type did not have scores above the recommended cut-off of 55.[59] These data suggest that high scores on the Brown ADD Scales may be helpful in identifying individuals who are likely to meet criteria for ADHD-inattentive, but that low scores on the Brown ADD Scales are less meaningful diagnostically.

The Brown ADD Scales are not *DSM-IV-TR* based, but a number of the *DSM-IV-TR* inattentive constructs are included. These scales are unique in their focus on executive functioning in the context of ADHD, but have very little information about hyperactivity and impulsivity. Although a collateral reporter may complete the adolescent forms, there are not specific normative data for interpreting parent and/or teacher ratings for this age group.

Overall, the Brown ADD Scales may be useful to expand understanding of executive deficits as part of an ADHD evaluation, particularly when forming an applied treatment plan. At this time, these scales have less utility in diagnostic formulation as executive deficits are not part of the *DSM-IV-TR* criteria for ADHD.

Useful resource

More information regarding test forms and manuals for the Brown ADD Scales can be found through the publisher at http://psychcorp.pearsonassessments.com.

Behavior Assessment System for Children, Second Edition

The Behavior Assessment System for Children, Second Edition (BASC-2)[28], is a broadband assessment tool that includes symptoms and associated signs of ADHD. Parent (parent rating scales [PRS]) and teacher forms (teacher rating scales [TRS]) can be used to describe patients aged 2–21 years. A self-report form (self-report of personality [SRP]) is available for patients 6 years old through college age. The BASC-2 Progress Monitors are a subset of BASC-2 items;

parent/teacher forms are available for rating students 2–21 years, and the self-report can be completed by students in 3rd to 12th grade. Parent and self-report forms are available in Spanish or English; teacher forms are available in English. The BASC-2 Progress Monitors were published in 2009, updating the BASC-Monitor.[60]

Structure and format
The TRS and PRS are each available for three different age levels (preschool, ages 2–5; child, ages 6–11; and adolescent, ages 12–21). The TRS has 100–139 items and the PRS has 134–160 items; length varies by age of child being rated. The SRP form is available for four different age levels (child interview, ages 6–7; child, ages 8–11; adolescent, ages 12–21; and post-secondary, ages 18–25); length ranges from 139–185 items. For children who are 6 or 7 years old, self-report is obtained with the SRP-Interview (SRP-I) form, by which children answer yes/no questions that are read aloud by the examiner.

The BASC-2 includes a number of adaptive and clinical scales, as well as validity indices and optional content scales. Various combinations of these scales are summarized by composite scores; there are five TRS and PRS composites: externalizing problems, internalizing problems, adaptive skills, school problems, and behavioral symptoms index; and five SRP composites: school problems, internalizing problems, inattention/hyperactivity, personal adjustment, and emotional symptoms index.

Note that the SRP and the observer-completed scales cover different content areas, with overlap for only six scales (anxiety, attention problems, atypicality, depression, hyperactivity, and somatization). Some scales vary by rater type and/or by age.

The BASC-2 Progress Monitor has a separate test administration form for each of four composite scales: externalizing and ADHD problems, internalizing problems, social withdrawal, and adaptive skills. Each form is available as a parent-, teacher-, or student-rated version, with parent and student forms in Spanish or English. Parent forms are further divided by age (preschool forms for 2–5 year olds; child/adolescent forms for kindergarten through to 12th grade). Each form has 15–20 items.

For all TRS, PRS, and SRP forms, and also the BASC-2 Progress Monitor, each item is rated on a 4-point frequency scale (N, never; S, sometimes; O, often; and A, almost always). The SRP also includes some true/false format items.

Scoring and interpretation
For all scoring modalities, each item response is converted to an item raw score of 0 (never) to 3 (almost always). Item scores for each scale are summed, then converted to a percentile and *T*-score for each scale using normative data stratified by age (2- to 3-year groupings for children and adolescents). The manual recommends use of the combined gender sample, but gender-specific norms are also provided.

High scores on the BASC-2 clinical scales and the four composite scores based on these scales indicate higher frequency of problem behaviors. The adaptive scales and the adaptive skills composite are interpreted in the opposite direction; high scores on the BASC-2 adaptive scales and/or the adaptive skills composite indicate intact functioning (low scores indicate areas of concern).

Pros, cons, and best uses
The BASC-2 has a very comprehensive manual that includes a full description of the normative samples and psychometric data. Certain scales on the BASC-2 have low discriminative powers; for example, the attention problems scale is elevated not only in the sample of children with ADHD, but also in clinical samples for mental retardation, depression, and bipolar disorder. However, data from the BASC-2 Progress Monitor support good discriminative validity (including differentiation between ADHD subtypes). As indicated by the scale name, the BASC-2 Progress Monitor is intended for monitoring progress rather than initial diagnosis. The BASC-2 is not *DSM-IV* based, but a number of relevant constructs are represented. The validity indices are a useful element on the BASC-2.

There is minimal overlap of scales across the three rater types, which makes integration of results more complex for interpretation. Interpretation varies for the clinical scales (and composites based on these scales) compared with the adaptive scales (and the adaptive skills composite); this is a possible source of interpretation errors. Be mindful that concerns are represented by high scores on the clinical components, and by low scores on the adaptive components.

Overall, the BASC-2 can be used to gather data about a number of different concerns, including those related to ADHD. Users should keep in mind that individual scales on the BASC-2 are not diagnosis specific, but describe general problems that can occur across a number of clinical conditions.

Useful resource
The BASC-2 is available from http://psychcorp.pearsonassessments.com.

Achenbach System of Empirically Based Assessment
The Achenbach System of Empirically Based Assessment (ASEBA) is a series of assessment tools that includes the well-known child behavior checklist (CBCL),[23,24] teacher report form (TRF), and youth self-report (YSR), as well as an adult behavior checklist (ABCL),[61] adult self-report (ASR), older adult behavior checklist (OABCL),[62] and older adult self-report (OASR). These are all broadband assessment tools that include constructs relevant to ADHD.

The CBCL is completed by parents, other close relatives, and/or guardians about children aged 1.5–18 years (preschool form, 1.5–5 years; school-age form, 6–18 years). The TRF is used for ratings of children aged 1.5–18 years by teachers (or caregivers for the caregiver-teacher report form, ages 1.5 –5 years). Youths aged 11–18 years old can complete the YSR. The ABCL (observer-completed [eg, spouse, partner]) and ASR (self-report) describe people aged

18–59 years old. The OABCL (observer-completed [eg, spouse, partner]) and OASR (self-report) describe people who are 60 years or older. The forms are available in a number of languages.

Structure and format

All of the ASEBA rating scale forms have randomly intermingled items that can be compiled to obtain the following common elements:

- syndromes: ie, statistically derived scales;
- *DSM*-oriented scales: contain items seen as being consistent with *DSM-IV* diagnostic categories, including an ADHD scale;
- composite scores: includes internalizing problems, externalizing problems, and total problems; and
- survey items: includes patient's disabilities and strengths, as well as the rater's primary concerns (these are not scored).

Each preschool form (parent form, CBCL/1.5–5/language developmental survey [LDS]; teacher form [C-TRF]) has 99 "problem items." The parent preschool form includes an optional LDS, which can be used with children who are 18–35 months old to capture data about expressive language and risk factors for language delays. This survey produces two percentiles for average length of phrases and vocabulary score.

The school-age forms (parent form, CBCL/6–18; TRF/6–18; YSR/11–18) begin with two pages to describe the child's activities, interpersonal relationships, and academic performance/placement; data from these pages are used to calculate competence, academic performance, and total adaptive functioning scores. For all school-aged forms, these pages are followed by 112 "problem items."

All "problem items" on the ASEBA scales are rated on a 3-point scale ranging from 0 "not true (as far as you know)" to 2 "very true or often true." The CBCL/6–18, YSR/11–18, and adult forms ask about the past 6 months. The preschool forms, TRF/6–18, and older adult forms ask about the past 2 months.

Scoring and interpretation

A multicultural option is available with the school-aged module, allowing comparison with normative samples from multiple cultures.[63] Ratings from up to eight forms (within the same age-bracket of forms) can be compared in a cross-informant report, including rankings on degree of agreement between informants.

Normative data are stratified by age and gender, leading to percentiles and *T*-scores. Diagnostic cut-off scores are also described, differentiating among "normal," "borderline clinical," and "clinical" ranges. Note that scoring updates were published for a number of the ASEBA forms in 2009; updated software is required to obtain some of the scores.

High scores on the syndrome scales, *DSM*-informed scales, and composite scores indicate higher levels of concern (ie, clinical classification likely). In contrast, high scores on the LDS scales, competence scales, positive qualities scale, adaptive functioning scales, and personal strengths scale indicate high levels of competence (ie, "normal" classification).

Pros, cons, and best uses

Overall, the ASEBA is a sophisticated instrument with a number of technical strengths. The ASEBA scales have a long history of use and research, and very good reliability and validity, including discriminative validity. The normative samples are extensive and well stratified by age, gender, and geographic region. Like the BASC-2, the ASEBA is not *DSM-IV* based, but includes items that are relevant to *DSM-IV* diagnoses. A number of scores can be obtained on the ASEBA forms. The ASEBA has the strongest multicultural presence of any scale reviewed in this publication, including research literature and alternate normative data samples.

Like the BASC-2, interpretation varies for high scores on various ASEBA scales; this is a possible source for examiner error in interpretation. Be attentive to the direction of each scale when interpreting *T*-scores. It may help to keep in mind the scale label – if it describes a desirable attribute, a high score is desired (and vice versa).

Useful resource

ASEBA components can be found at www.aseba.org.

Rating scales for adults

The past 10 years have seen a substantial increase in the recognition of ADHD in adults. Consistent with longitudinal studies that have estimated that approximately half of children and adolescents with ADHD will continue to experience symptoms and impairment into adulthood, recent prevalence estimates for adult ADHD indicate that 4.4–5.2% of adults in the US meet criteria for the disorder.[2–5] Fortunately, along with the increase in recognition of the disorder in adults, there has also been an increase in the tools that can be used to assess ADHD and monitor outcomes. The remainder of this section will describe and evaluate a range of scales used to assess ADHD and related impairments in adults. A summary of these instruments is shown in Table 4. It should be noted that the list of rating scales described here is not exhaustive. Rather, those scales that are most widely used and represented in the relevant clinical literature were included. Also, many scales that have been used in the assessment of adults with ADHD but do not focus on primary symptoms and impairments (ie, scales measuring mood problems or substance use) are not included in this discussion.

At least six separate scales have been used with some frequency to assess the signs and symptoms of ADHD (Table 4).

Table 4 Summary of rating scales used to assess ADHD and related impairments in adults

Scale Name	Source	Rater types	*DSM-IV* symptoms represented?	Norma-tive data?	Psychometric properties	Notes
Adult ADHD Self-Report Scale (ASRS)	Available for free in public domain	Self-report	Partially	No	Demonstrated specificity and sensitivity for identifying potential ADHD	Functions well as a screening instrument
ADHD Rating Scale-IV (ADHD-RS-IV)	Com-mercially available	Self-report, clinician	Yes	Not for adults	None established for adults	Lists all 18 *DSM-IV* symptoms
Adult ADHD Investigator Symptom Rating Scale (AISRS)	Not available publicly; may be available from developers	Designed to be administered by trained raters with specific educational require-ments	Yes	No	Empirically derived factor structure; demonstrated reliability and validity	Similar to ADHD-RS-IV, except uses specific prompts to probe symp-toms in adults
Brown ADD Scales for Adults	Com-mercially available from PsychCorp	Self-report	Not explicitly	Yes	Not reported or available	Emphasizes assessment of executive functioning
Conners' Adult ADHD Rating Scales (CAARS)	Com-mercially available	Self-report, observer, investigator	Yes	Yes, age- and gender-based	Empirically derived factor structure; demonstrated validity and reliability	Includes short and screening forms
Wender Utah Rating Scale (WURS)	Available for free in public domain	Self-report	Not explicitly	No	Empirically derived factor structure; demonstrated reliability and validity	Designed to assess childhood symptoms in adults; cut score used to adequately classify patients and non-patients

Adapted from Kessler et al;[64] Dupaul et al;[26] Spencer et al;[65] Brown et al;[29] Conners et al;[66] and Ward et al.[67]

ADHD Rating Scale-IV

The ADHD Rating Scale-IV (ADHD-RS-IV) was initially developed for use by parents and teachers to rate children and adolescents aged 5–17 years of age (please see page 17).[26] However, the scale has been adapted for use in several clinical trials of adults with ADHD to monitor treatment outcome.[68]

Structure and format
The ADHD-RS-IV contains the 18 *DSM-IV-TR* symptoms from criterion A (see Table 1);
9 inattentive and 9 hyperactive/impulsive symptoms.[1] Each symptom is rated on a 4-point
scale from 0 to 3, with 3 indicating severe. As such, total scores can range from 0 to 54.
The scale can be completed by a patient or observer (eg, spouse), as well as via clinical
interviewing by a clinician.

Scoring and interpretation
Scores are simply the total score across all 18 symptoms. Subscale scores for the 9 inattentive
and 9 hyperactive/impulsive symptoms (the range is 0–27 for each) can also be examined.
There are no established cut points for adults, although some studies have used scores above
22 or 24 as inclusion criteria. While there are normative data and scoring profiles for parent and
teacher ratings of children and adolescents, no such data are available for adults or for clinician-
completed forms.

Pros, cons, and best uses
The ADHD-RS-IV is simple and easy to use. It is also face valid since it simply lists the 18 *DSM-IV*
symptoms. The scale has been shown to be sensitive to the effects of treatment in adults[68]
and can be used either as a self-report instrument or by a clinician.[69] Its use in adults, however,
has not been extensively studied and its psychometric properties in this age group are not
well-established. This scale is probably best used to monitor symptom change as a function of
treatment instead of as a diagnostic tool in and of itself.

Adult ADHD Self-Report Scale
The Adult ADHD Self-Report Scale (ASRS) was developed by academic clinicians to be used
in clinical practice as a screening instrument for adult patients aged 18 years or older with
suspected ADHD.[64] Its use as a screening tool has been well established with 80% sensitivity
and 70% specificity.[64,70,71]

Structure and format
As expected with a screening tool, the ASRS is short; there are only six items each rated on a
5-point frequency scale. Though not explicitly analogous to *DSM-IV* symptoms, the six items
correspond to several of the ADHD symptoms. The scale is designed to be completed by
the patient.

Scoring and interpretation
Each item is scored as either 1 or 0, depending on the patient rating of each item (ranging from
"never" to "very often"). A total score of 4 or higher is deemed a positive score and is suggestive

of a full diagnosis. The ASRS is designed specifically as a screening instrument and a positive score suggests that further evaluation is necessary to fully assess ADHD.

Pros, cons, and best uses

As a screening instrument, the ASRS functions very well. It should not be used in any other capacity though, since it does not cover the full range of *DSM-IV* ADHD symptoms. The best use for this instrument is for busy primary care clinicians who need a quick and efficient way to screen for adult ADHD prior to additional evaluation or referral.

Useful resource

More information regarding the ASRS can be found at www.hcp.med.harvard.edu/ncs/asrs.php.

Adult ADHD Investigator Symptom Rating Scale

The Adult ADHD Investigator Symptom Rating Scale (AISRS) was developed to provide a more developmentally sensitive measure for adult ADHD, where symptoms may manifest themselves in unique ways compared to more traditional pediatric clinical presentations.[65,72] Its intended use is with patients 18 years of age and older.

Structure and format

The AISRS is designed to be administered in a semi-structured format by a trained clinician. Each of the 18 *DSM-IV* ADHD symptoms is reviewed, but in addition to asking questions verbatim, clinicians are trained to use symptom-specific probes to more accurately assess the adult manifestation of the disorder.

Scoring and interpretation

Each of the 18 items on the AISRS is rated by the clinician on a 4-point scale that ranges from 0–3. As such, the range of scores is similar to the ADHD-RS-IV. Interpretation of the AISRS scale is straightforward since higher scores reflect higher symptom counts. AISRS scores have been shown to be associated in an expected way with clinician ratings of functional impairment.[65]

Pros, cons, and best uses

The AISRS has been shown to be reliable, valid, and sensitive to treatment effects. It has been used in a number of clinical trials and has an empirically derived factor structure.[65,73,74] Critically, the instrument is developmentally sensitive to the adult manifestations of ADHD.[65] This rating scale does not appear to be available to the public, which is most likely due to its requirement of training in the use of the prompts and interview format; also, the scale does not have an accompanying manual. As such, the best uses for this instrument currently seem to be in the context of clinical trials, where raters can be explicitly trained in the application of the scale.

Brown ADD Scales for Adults

The Brown ADD Scales for Adults[29] are designed to assess associated signs of ADHD, specifically those in the area of executive functioning, such as organization and prioritization, working memory, processing speed, and multitasking. The scale was developed based on a conceptual model developed by the main author of the scales. The adult version of the Brown ADD Scales is designed to be used in individuals aged 18 year and older. Please see page 23 regarding the Brown ADD Scales for child/adolescent patients.

Structure and format

The Brown ADD Scales for Adults contains 40 items that yield five rationally derived cluster scores, focusing on different components of executive functioning. The scale is designed to be completed by the patient.

Scoring and interpretation

Raw scores from each of the clusters on the Brown ADD Scales for Adults, along with the total composite score are converted to *T*-scores. Normative data are available for this instrument, along with clinical recommendations for how to interpret scoring. Since the items do not reflect the specific *DSM-IV* diagnostic criteria for ADHD, however, the utility of the Brown ADD Scales for Adults as a diagnostic instrument is limited.

Pros, cons, and best uses

A few published studies have used the Brown ADD Scales to measure outcome for focused interventions targeting executive functioning in adults with ADHD; results suggest that there is treatment sensitivity for such types of interventions.[75,76] The adult form includes items about impact of ADHD in an academic setting; while this is useful for adults currently enrolled in classes, it is less relevant for adults in the workplace.

The Brown ADD Scales for Adults is relatively easy to use and assesses a domain of functioning not fully addressed by other assessment instruments. The Brown ADD Scales for Adults cannot really be used as a diagnostic tool or aid given its content. The best use for the scale at this time is probably as a way to identify individual treatment targets and/or to monitor such outcomes during the course of treatment.

Useful resource

More information regarding test forms and manuals for the Brown ADD Scales for Adults can be found through the publisher, http://psychcorp.pearsonassessments.com.

Conners' Adult ADHD Rating Scales

The Conners' Adult ADHD Rating Scales (CAARS) were first published in the late 1990s to complement the well-known set of child and adolescent rating scales that had been in use for several decades prior to that point.[66] The scales offer several different forms that can be used for different purposes. The CAARS is intended for use in individuals aged 18 years and older.

Structure and format

The CAARS has six different formats; three formats designed for self-report and three for observer report. The long versions contain 66 items each, grouped into four empirically derived factors, plus an ADHD index, and subscales that represent the *DSM-IV* inattention, hyperactivity/impulsivity, and total symptoms. The short and screening forms contain fewer items and subscales, but both still contain the ADHD index and *DSM-IV* subscales. Several clinical trials have also used an investigator version of the CAARS (CAARS-INV).[77,78] This is not a separate form, but simply an observer form that is administered in interview format by a trained clinician-investigator. The CAARS has been widely used and demonstrates good psychometric properties, including high reliability and validity.[66]

Scoring and interpretation

Each item on the CAARS forms is scored on a 4-point scale, from 0 to 3. Factor/subscale scores are derived separately and converted to *T*-scores, which are based on age and gender norms. The ADHD index is used as a reliable and valid predictor of ADHD status, and this subscale is present across different versions of the scale.

Pros, cons, and best uses

The CAARS scales have a number of strengths. They have been widely used and validated, have more extensive norms than any other adult ADHD rating scale, and have been shown to be sensitive to the effects of different treatments. The different forms allow clinicians to select which form is most appropriate for use. Long versions of the CAARS can be used in initial diagnostic assessment to determine norm-based levels of symptoms from both the patient and an observer. The short and screening versions can be used to determine the need for additional assessment or to monitor treatment progress across time.

Useful resource
Further information regarding the CAARS can be found at www.mhs.com.

Wender Utah Rating Scale

The Wender Utah Rating Scale (WURS) was developed more than 15 years ago to assess the retrospective symptoms of ADHD in adults presenting for assessment in adulthood.[67] This scale was the first designed to be used explicitly with adult patients suspected of having ADHD. It is not linked to *DSM-IV* criteria, which were not published until 1994. The main focus of the WURS is to retrospectively assess the presence of childhood symptoms in adult patients.

Structure and format

The WURS consists of 61 items that are rated on a 5-point scale from 0 to 4. Each item asks about whether a particular symptom or behavior was present during childhood. Patients rate the frequency with which each item described them as children.

Scoring and interpretation

A subset of 25 of the 61 questions is explicitly associated with ADHD. The minimum score of these items is 0 and the maximum score is 100. The original article determined that a cut-off score of 46 across these 25 items was best to differentiate those with and without adult ADHD.[67]

Pros, cons, and best uses

The WURS has been relatively widely used and has demonstrated good psychometric properties (ie, factor structure, reliability).[79,80] Of all available instruments with self-report measures, the WURS is the most comprehensive with respect to assessing childhood symptoms. The instrument is not concordant with current *DSM-IV* symptom criteria and does not assess current symptoms or impairment in adult patients. Its best use is to aid in a more comprehensive assessment of ADHD by providing objective measures of childhood symptomatology and functioning.

Scales used to assess ADHD-related impairment and quality of life

Several scales have been developed in recent years to measure the problems that ADHD causes in day-to-day functioning, whether expressed in terms of impairment or quality of life (QoL) (Table 5). Several studies have documented that the symptoms of ADHD can severely impact QoL throughout the lifespan,[90-92] and that QoL is often correlated with severity of ADHD symptoms.[93] Assessing impairment is critical, not only to establish the initial diagnosis of ADHD, but also when monitoring response to treatment.[94] Pharmaceutical studies now require assessment of QoL among the patient-reported outcome measures.[95,96]

ADHD Impact Module

The ADHD Impact Module (AIM) was developed to assess the health-related QoL (HRQoL) in people with ADHD. It is available for completion by parents about children (AIM-C)[72] and for self-report by adults (AIM-A).[81]

Table 5 Summary of rating scales used to assess impairment and quality of life in ADHD

Scale Name	Source	Rater types	Child or adolescent	Adult	Normative data	Psychometric properties	Notes
ADHD Impact Module for Adults (AIM-A)	Available from publisher	Self-report	X	✓	No	Demonstrated reliability; validity	ADHD-specific
ADHD Impact Module for Children (AIM-C)	Available from publisher	Parent	✓	X	No	Demonstrated reliability; validity	ADHD-specific
Adult ADHD Quality of Life Scale (AAQoL)	Available from developers	Self-report	X	✓	No	None published	ADHD-specific
Child Health and Illness Profile, Adolescent Edition (CHIP-AE)	Available from developers	Self-report 11–17 years	✓	X	Yes	Demonstrated reliability; validity	Generic QoL measure
Child Health and Illness Profile, Children Edition (CHIP-CE)	Available from developers	Parent or self-report 6–11 years	✓	X	Yes	Demonstrated reliability; validity	Generic QoL measure; demonstrated treatment sensitivity for ADHD
Children's Health Questionnaire (CHQ)	Available from publisher	Parent and self-report forms	✓	X	Yes	Manual notes acceptable psychometrics, though not published	Generic QoL measure; demonstrated treatment sensitivity for ADHD
Pediatric Quality of Life Inventory (PedsQL)	Available from one distributor	Parent and self-report forms	✓	X	Yes	Demonstrated reliability; validity	Generic QoL measure; preliminary data suggest treatment sensitivity for ADHD
Weiss Functional Impairment Rating Scale, Parent Report (WFIRS-P)	Available from developers	Parent	✓	X	No	Instructions note good reliability and validity, though not published	ADHD-specific; designed to evaluate functional impairment of ADHD
Weiss Functional Impairment Rating Scale, Self-Report (WFIRS-S)	Available from developers	Self-report	X	✓	No	Instructions note good reliability and validity, though not published	ADHD-specific; designed to evaluate functional impairment of ADHD
Youth Quality of Life Instrument (YQoL)	Available from developers	Self-report	✓	X	No	Demonstrated reliability; validity	Generic QoL measure

QoL, quality of life. Adapted from Landgraf;[81] Landgraf et al;[72] Brod et al;[82] Starfield et al;[83] Riley et al;[84] Landgraf et al;[85] Varni et al;[86] Weiss et al;[87] Weiss;[88] and Patrick et al.[89]

Structure and format
The AIM-C has two core scales describing the impact of ADHD on the child (eight items) and on home life/family (10 items). There are several items regarding medications, variability across the day, cooperation from the child's school, and economic impact of ADHD symptoms. The AIM-C has been shown to be sensitive to treatment effects[97] and has demonstrated reliability and validity.[72]

The AIM-A contains 57 items that are rationally divided into six separate subscales. In addition, several global impact questions are included, along with several questions on the impact of ADHD on work and economic functioning. The AIM-A has been shown to be sensitive to treatment effects in several randomized clinical trials and has demonstrated reliability and validity.[81, 98,99]

Scoring and interpretation
Each of the items on the AIM is scored using a Likert scale wherein raters are asked how much they agree or disagree with a range of statements or how well each statement describes the patient. The Likert responses are then summed and used to determine across the domains of functioning how significantly ADHD is impacting the patient's day-to-day functioning and QoL.

Pros, cons, and best uses
The AIM-C and AIM-A cover a wide range of domains of functioning. Their best uses are to document impairment required to make an initial diagnosis of ADHD, and monitor individual treatment progress.

Useful resource
Further information about the AIM-C and AIM-A can be found at www.healthact.com/surveys.html.

Adult ADHD Quality of Life Scale
The Adult ADHD Quality of Life Scale (AAQoL) was developed to measure the extent to which ADHD impacts functioning across domains in adults with ADHD.[82]

Structure and format
The AAQoL contains 29 items that form four empirically derived factors covering different domains of functioning. The scale has been shown to have good factor structure, reliability, and validity.[82] The AAQoL has also been shown to be sensitive to the effects of treatment in several different studies.[100]

Scoring and interpretation
Each of the items on the AAQoL is scored on a 5-point scale from 1 to 5. A total score is derived, along with subscale scores for each of the four factors.

Pros, cons, and best uses
Similar to the AIM-A, the AAQoL is a useful tool in studies or in clinical practice. The scale does not appear to be commercially available. If available, the AAQoL could be used to help assess initial impairment or to monitor treatment progress.

Child Health and Illness Profile
The Child Health and Illness Profile (CHIP) is a set of generic QoL instruments that have been used in ADHD research. It is available in a child edition (CHIP-CE, 6–11 years old)[84] for parent- or self-report, and an adolescent edition (CHIP-AE, 11–17 years old)[83] for self-report.

Structure and format
The CHIP-CE has 45 items divided into four domains: satisfaction, comfort, resilience, and risk avoidance. The CHIP-AE has 108 items in these same four domains, as well as achievement and optional "disorders" domains. Each item is rated on a 5-point scale; the CHIP-CE child-report form uses cartoons and graduated-circle response options to help children understand the rating options. The CHIP-CE has good psychometric properties,[101–103] and has demonstrated treatment sensitivity for ADHD in children.[104] The CHIP-AE also has established psychometric properties.[105,106]

Scoring and interpretation
Computerized scoring produces a *T*-score for each domain, based on the normative sample for each CHIP measure. High scores on the CHIP indicate good health in that domain; *T*-scores that are 43 or lower indicate poor health.

Pros, cons, and best uses
The CHIP instruments are not specific to ADHD, but help describe impairment that may be related to symptoms of ADHD. They can be used to document impairment for initial diagnosis of ADHD and monitor change in impairment during treatment.

> **Useful resource**
> The CHIP instruments are available from Johns Hopkins School of Public Health at http://childhealthprofile.org.

Child Health Questionnaire
The Child Health Questionnaire (CHQ) is a generic QoL instrument that has been used extensively in ADHD research. It is available in short (28 items) and full-length (50 items) forms for completion by parents about children aged 5–18 years, as well as in a self-report form (87 items) for completion by children aged 10–18 years.[85]

Structure and format

The CHQ includes two main clusters of items: physical and psychosocial health. Each item is rated on a Likert scale, describing the degree of limitation, satisfaction, frequency, or severity. The psychosocial items from the CHQ have been shown to be sensitive to treatment effects in ADHD.[107] The manual reports acceptable psychometric properties.

Scoring and interpretation

Separate scores are available for the physical items and the psychosocial items; a combined score is also available. These scores can be used to describe the child's QoL and impairment related to ADHD symptoms.

Pros, cons, and best uses

The CHQ is not specific to ADHD, but describes a number of ways ADHD symptoms can impact functioning. It can be used to document impairment for initial diagnosis of ADHD and monitor change in impairment during treatment.

Useful resource

Further information about the CHQ can be found at www.healthact.com/surveys-chq.php.

Pediatric Quality of Life Inventory

The Pediatric Quality of Life Inventory (PedsQL) is a modular system for assessing health-related quality of life (HRQoL) in children and adolescents.[86] The PedsQL instruments, while not specific to ADHD, can help describe impairment possibly due to ADHD symptoms. The standard form includes generic core scales; there are optional condition-specific modules (eg, asthma, arthritis, cancer). The self-report form can be completed by 5–18 year olds, with separate forms for each age group (5–7, 8–12, 13–18 years). Parent forms are available to describe 2–18 year olds (divided into developmentally appropriate forms: 2–4, 5–7, 8–12, and 13–18 years).

Structure and format

The generic PedsQL has 23 items divided into four core domains: physical functioning, emotional functioning, social functioning, and school functioning. There is also a 15-item short form. For most forms, each item is rated on a 5-point scale ranging from 0 ("never") to 4 ("almost always"). The self-report form for 5–7 year olds uses a 3-point scale with faces to anchor each rating. There are two standard time frames for report: past month or past 7 days. The PedsQL has good psychometric properties.[86,108,109] It has been demonstrated as useful in documenting lower HRQoL in children with ADHD,[92,110] and preliminary data suggest treatment sensitivity.[55]

Scoring and interpretation

Each item is transformed into a 0–100 scale, with a rating of 0 becoming an item score of 100 (ie, 1=75, 2=50, 3=25, and 4=0). A mean scale score is calculated for each of the four domains. A physical health summary score is the average physical functioning scale score. A psychosocial health summary score is calculated by finding the average of items from the other three scales. The mean score for all items on the generic core PedsQL is the total scale score. Normative data are available for comparison. Higher scores on the PedsQL indicate better HRQoL.

Pros, cons, and best uses

The instruments can be used to document impairment for initial diagnosis of ADHD and monitor change in impairment during treatment.

Useful resource

The PedsQL forms are licensed for use through www.mapi-trust.org. Administration and scoring instructions are available from the author's website, http://pedsql.org.

Weiss Functional Impairment Rating Scale

The Weiss Functional Impairment Rating Scale (WFIRS) is available for completion by parents whose children have ADHD (WFIRS-P)[87] or for self-report by adults with ADHD (WIFRS-S).[88] The WFIRS scales measure functional impairment, which some could argue is a distinct construct from QoL. Broadly speaking, though, the WFIRS-S, like the other scales, measures the extent to which having ADHD impacts day-to-day functioning in the lives of affected adults.

Structure and format

The WFIRS-P contains 50 items divided into six domains: family, learning and school, life skills, child's self-concept, social activities, and risky activities. The WIFRS-S contains 69 items divided into seven domains: family, work, school, life skills, self-concept, social, and risk. The WFIRS-P has demonstrated treatment sensitivity;[111] no psychometric data are currently available for review. However, studies are underway to evaluate the psychometric properties of the WFIRS-S.

Scoring and interpretation

Each of the items on the WFIRS-S is scored on a 4-point scale from 0 to 3. Subscale scores are then derived for each domain of functioning as well as a total score. Individual items that are rated "2" or "3" are considered "impaired." Scoring instructions suggest reporting a domain as "impaired" if at least one item is rated "3" *or* at least two items are rated "2" or higher.

Pros, cons, and best uses
The WFIRS represents an attempt to document the kinds of idiosyncratic problems that adults with ADHD experience on a day-to-day basis. The domains of functioning are comprehensive and intuitive. The psychometric properties of the WFIRS are not yet published; early studies suggest good sensitivity to treatment effects (at least for the WFIRS-P). If good psychometric properties can be demonstrated, the WFIRS will be a useful instrument both in the initial diagnostic assessment process and for monitoring ongoing treatment.

Youth Quality of Life Instruments
Like the PedsQL, the Youth Quality of Life instruments (YQoL)[89] are a modular system with generic and condition-specific modules. The YQoL is designed for self-report by adolescents, 11–18 years old. It is available in a surveillance version (YQoL-S) for use in brief surveys and a research version (YQoL-R) for more in-depth HRQoL information.

Structure and format
The YQoL-R has 57 items to assess HRQoL for the present day, including four domains: sense of self, social relationships, culture and community, and general QoL. The YQoL-S has 13 items; it is not divided into domains. Each item is rated on a 5-point scale ranging from 0 ("never") to 4 ("very often"). Both modules have "contextual" items that can be verified by an observer and "perceptual" items that can only be obtained by self-report. Acceptable psychometrics have been documented.[89] The YQoL has been used to show lower HRQoL in adolescents with ADHD,[112] but no data have been published to date regarding treatment sensitivity for ADHD.

Scoring and interpretation
A total score can be obtained for the YQoL-R, as well as separate domain scores. Each score is reported using a 0–100 scale; higher scores on the YQoL indicate better HRQoL.

Pros, cons, and best uses
The YQoL instruments are not specific to ADHD, but help describe impairment that may be secondary to symptoms of ADHD. They can be used to document impairment for initial diagnosis of ADHD and monitor change in impairment during treatment.

Useful resource
Information is available on the YQoL developer's website, www.seaqolgroup.org.

3 Structured interviews and questionnaires for assessing ADHD

As noted in Chapter 1, the cornerstone for a good clinical evaluation of ADHD is the clinical interview. The interview should integrate information from the rating scales and other data collected from the patient or the patient's caregiver to confirm that each of the diagnostic criteria have been met. The combination of structured and semi-structured interviews provides the most efficient means of gathering information about the presentation of ADHD symptoms, the impairment they cause, the duration and severity of the symptoms, and the potential presence of other problems that may better account for the symptoms.

In general, a structured interview is clearly scripted, with yes/no decision points that lead to skipping sections or continuing with more detailed items. In contrast, a semi-structured interview provides a general structure for an experienced clinician to follow in exploring diagnostic possibilities. Semi-structured interviews usually require the clinician to probe or investigate with questions beyond those on the printed page (or computer screen). Structured interviews have advantages in that they can be administered by a technician, or even completed by the patient/caregiver in some instances; semi-structured interviews generally require clinical background and training.

Interviews and questionnaires for children and adolescents

Some of the following interviews are modular, allowing the clinician to administer only the sections relevant to his or her questions about a child (Table 6). The primary function of broad interviews such as those described below in the context of an ADHD evaluation is to examine differential diagnostic possibilities and comorbidities. Disorders that are endorsed should be explored further in a clinician-based interview; results from a single instrument cannot substitute for a clinical evaluation.[117]

Diagnostic Interview Schedule for Children-IV
The National Institute of Mental Health's Diagnostic Interview Schedule for Children Version IV (DISC-IV)[114] is a structured clinical interview that covers the most common psychiatric disorders in children and adolescents. The DISC-IV is designed to be administered by a clinician, technician, or research assistant. The computerized version of the DISC-IV can also be completed by an adolescent (DISC-A, for adolescents aged 9–17 years) or a parent/caregiver (DISC-P, for caregivers of children aged 6–17 years). It is available in multiple languages.

Table 6 Summary of interviews used to assess ADHD and related impairments in children and adolescents

Interview name	Source	Age range	Time to administer	Type of interview	DSM-IV-TR basis?	Psychometric properties	Notes
Conners–March Developmental Questionnaire (CMDQ)	Commercially available from the publisher	3–17 years	20 mins	General; semi-structured	X	Not applicable—does not provide a diagnosis	Paper–pencil measure; can be completed by parent/caregiver as a questionnaire or by clinician during interview with parent/caregiver
Diagnostic Interview Schedule for Children-IV (DISC-IV)	Available from the developers	6–17 years (9–17 years for self-report)	45–90 mins	Comprehensive; structured	✓	Based on studies of past versions of the DISC; further study needed with DISC-IV	Computerized; can be completed by patient, parent; can be administered by clinician as a computerized interview
Diagnostic Interview for Children and Adolescents-IV (DICA-IV)	Commercially available from the publisher	6–17 years (13–17 years for self-report)	5–20 mins per category (60 min average)	Comprehensive; structured	✓	Based on studies of past versions of the DICA; further study needed with DICA-IV	Computerized; can be completed by patient, parent; can be administered by clinician as a computerized interview. Critical items list helps screen for high-risk behaviors
Schedule for Affective Disorders and Schizophrenia for School-Age Children (Kiddie-SADS, or K-SADS)	Available from the developers	6–17 years	30–90 mins	Comprehensive; semi-structured	✓	Preliminary findings suggest good test-retest reliability and construct validity	Paper–pencil measure; clinician must be trained to administer; clinician-administered to parent and patient

Adapted from Conners et al;[113] Shaffer et al;[114] Reich et al;[115] and Kaufman et al.[116]

The DISC-IV has six major sections and is divided into 24 diagnostic modules (including a module for ADHD), each of which can be administered independently. The DISC-IV can be used to gather information about symptoms in the past 4 weeks, past 12 months, and "whole life" (ie, since 5 years old). The interview takes approximately 45–90 minutes to administer.

The DISC-IV has grown from a long history of research-based interviews. Test–retest reliability is acceptable for most diagnoses, with parent results showing greater reliability than self-report. The DISC-IV is typically used in research settings, and sometimes for screening large populations (eg, juvenile justice system) to identify which children require a clinical evaluation. It is thorough, but lengthy.

Useful resource

The DISC-IV can be obtained through Columbia University, disc@childpsych.columbia.edu.

Diagnostic Interview for Children and Adolescents-IV

The Diagnostic Interview for Children and Adolescents-IV (DICA-IV) is a comprehensive, structured, *DSM-IV*-based interview.[115] The DICA-IV can be completed by children 6–12 years old (child form), adolescents 13–17 years old (adolescent form), or parents/caregivers of 6- to 17-year-old children/adolescents. The parent version includes items about prenatal, perinatal, and early childhood development. When administered by an experienced clinician, probing is encouraged in determining the presence/absence of symptoms. The DICA-IV has a 4th grade reading level, and has been translated into many languages.

The DICA-IV is divided into 28 categories (including a category for ADHD), each of which can be administered independently. Each category takes approximately 5–20 minutes to administer; an average interview takes about 60 minutes. High-risk features, such as suicidal ideation, violent tendencies, and drug use, are identified on the "Stein-Reich Critical Items" listing. This interview gathers information about lifetime history of diagnoses.

As with the DISC, the DICA-IV is the latest generation of an interview with a long history. Previous versions of the DICA have good psychometric properties. Limited research publications with the DICA-IV indicate reasonable reliability, with better reliability for internalizing disorders and for adolescents (as opposed to externalizing disorders and children).[118] The DICA-IV has been used in a number of epidemiological studies and is often used to establish entry criteria for other studies.

Useful resource

The DICA-IV can be found at www.mhs.com.

Schedule for Affective Disorders and Schizophrenia for School-Age Children

There are a number of versions of the Schedule for Affective Disorders and Schizophrenia for School-Age Children (Kiddie-SADs or K-SADS) in use; the most current at the time this text was prepared is the Present and Lifetime Version (K-SADS-PL).[116] This semi-structured interview can be used to rate severity of symptoms while assessing current and lifetime history of a number of *DSM-IV* disorders (including ADHD). It is designed for use with 6- to 17-year-old children/adolescents; a preschool version of the K-SADS-PL is currently being investigated.[119] It is available in many languages, but must be administered by a clinician with specialized training in the K-SADS-PL.

As a semi-structured interview, the probes listed are suggested ways to obtain relevant information for each item; the interviewer should use language that is appropriate for the setting. Interviews should be conducted with parent(s) and with child; the final ratings incorporate all sources of information. Adolescents are usually interviewed before their parent(s); the opposite order is recommended for younger patients. Discrepancies are resolved using further queries and clinical judgment.

A typical administration of the K-SADS begins with a 10- to 15-minute unstructured interview, followed by a screening interview that identifies which of 20 diagnostic areas to investigate further. Responses during these sections determine which of the five supplements are administered (eg, behavioral disorder supplement, which includes ADHD) and the sequence of these supplements. The clinician summarizes all information with the "Summary Lifetime Diagnoses Checklist" and "Children's Global Assessment Scales". A typical K-SADS interview lasts 30–60 minutes.

In general, psychometrics for the K-SADS-PL are reasonable. Test–retest reliability is good for current diagnoses, and slightly better for lifetime diagnoses (particularly for affective disorders, CD, and ODD), with ADHD reliability falling in the reasonable range.[120]

Useful resource

The K-SADS-PL may be obtained from the primary author's website, www.wpic.pitt.edu/ksads

---

Conners–March Developmental Questionnaire

The Conners–March Developmental Questionnaire (CMDQ)[113] can be administered as a semi-structured interview or as a questionnaire to gather a detailed patient history about a 3- to 17-year-old child/adolescent. It is completed by the parent/caregiver (or by the clinician during an interview with the parent/caregiver). While not limited to ADHD, the items obtain information that is important to review in the context of an ADHD evaluation.

Information obtained with the CMDQ includes: demographic information about patient and family, school information (locations, performance, behavior), family medical history, psychiatric medication history, therapy history, pregnancy and birth history, developmental/temperament history, family psychiatric history, and medical history of the child. The CMDQ takes about 20 minutes to complete.

The parent-completed CMDQ is an efficient way to gather data. It can be mailed to parents and completed before they come for their first visit, or it can be given to the parent(s) during the first session to complete.

Useful resource
The CMDQ can be found at www.mhs.com.

Interviews and questionnaires for adults

Diagnosis of ADHD in adulthood is challenging since the *DSM-IV* criteria were developed for pediatric populations and were not formally evaluated in individuals older than 17 years of age. As such, having a systematic approach for assessing and diagnosing the disorder is critical. The rating scales discussed in Chapter 2 can be useful for evaluating the signs and symptoms of ADHD, or for assessing the impact that the disorder has on day-to-day functioning. However, more information must be collected in order to ensure that all of the criteria for diagnosis are met. To date, there are only two semi-structured interviews used explicitly for diagnosis of ADHD in adults, which are listed in Table 7.

Adult ADHD Clinician Diagnostic Scale

The Adult ADHD Clinician Diagnostic Scale (ACDS) is a semi-structured interview designed to be administered by trained clinicians.[121,123] The interview includes items from the ADHD-RS-IV as well the items and probes from the AISRS. As such, the ACDS is designed to provide developmentally sensitive probes for evaluating symptoms of ADHD in adulthood. The ACDS

Table 7 Summary of diagnostic interviews used to assess ADHD and related impairments in adults

Interview name	Source	Format	DSM-IV criteria covered?	Psychometric properties	Notes
Adult ADHD Clinician Diagnostic Scale (ACDS)	Does not appear to be available publicly; may be available from developers	Semi-structured	Partially	None established for adults	Has been used in a number of clinical trials for adults; uses similar prompts as AISRS
Conners' Adult ADHD Diagnostic Interview for *DSM-IV* (CAADID)	Commercially available from a variety of sources	Semi-structured	Yes	Demonstrated validity and reliability	Explicitly covers all 5 *DSM-IV* diagnostic criteria; includes a history section to review additional clinical information

AISRS, Adult ADHD Investigator Symptom Rating Scale; *DSM-IV, Diagnostic and Statistical Manual of Mental Disorders,* (Fourth Edition). Adapted from Adler et al;[121] and Epstein et al.[122]

has been used in several clinical trials for treatment of ADHD in adults.[124,125] The ACDS has also been used in several epidemiological studies of prevalence rates of adult ADHD in the US and other countries.[2,4]

At present, the ACDS does not appear to be commercially available, though it may be attainable directly from the developers. Studies that have used the instrument have generally required extensive training on its use. The psychometric properties of the ACDS have not been published. Though used in academic settings and clinical trials, the ACDS does not appear to be a readily available instrument for clinicians at present.

Conners' Adult ADHD Diagnostic Interview for *DSM-IV*

The Conners' Adult ADHD Diagnostic Interview for *DSM-IV* (CAADID) is designed to explicitly cover each of the five *DSM-IV* criteria in a semi-structured interview format.[122] The CAADID also includes a background and history section in addition to the diagnostic criteria. This section can be completed by the patient as a questionnaire or by the clinician in interview format. The background section allows the collection of a range of other relevant clinical information (eg, developmental and educational history, medical history, substance use history) that can help to inform differential diagnosis. In the section reviewing diagnostic criteria, the CAADID explicitly reviews each of the 18 *DSM-IV* symptoms and queries about their presence in both adulthood and childhood. Like the ACDS and the AISRS, the CAADID offers a range of prompts that can be used by the clinician to assess symptoms. A number of questions regarding chronicity, pervasiveness, impairment, and age of onset of symptoms are also included to help determine the presence of additional *DSM-IV* criteria.

The CAADID has demonstrated good psychometric properties, including reliability and validity.[126] The CAADID has also been used in several large-scale clinical trials of treatment for adult ADHD.[124] One aspect of the CAADID that deserves mention is that it does not formally include extensive questions pertaining to the assessment of additional psychopathology. As such, in order to accurately rule out other disorders (per *DSM-IV* Criterion E), it is critical that users of the CAADID employ some kind of additional assessment measures to make a proper differential diagnosis. In spite of this limitation, the CAADID is a useful clinical instrument given its demonstrated psychometric properties, its availability, and its adherence to *DSM-IV* criteria.

> **Useful resource**
> More information regarding the CAADID can be found at www.mhs.com.

References

1. American Psychiatric Association. *Diagnostic and Statistical Manual of Mental Disorders.* 4th edn. Text Revision. Washington, DC: American Psychiatric Association; 2000.

2. Fayyad J, De Graaf R, Kessler R, et al. Cross-national prevalence and correlates of adult attention-deficit hyperactivity disorder. *Br J Psychiatry.* 2007;190:402-409.

3. Froehlich TE, Lanphear BP, Epstein JN, Barbaresi WJ, Katusic SK, Kahn RS. Prevalence, recognition, and treatment of attention-deficit/hyperactivity disorder in a national sample of US children. *Arch Pediatr Adolesc Med.* 2007;161:857-864.

4. Kessler RC, Adler L, Barkley R, et al. The prevalence and correlates of adult ADHD in the United States: results from the National Comorbidity Survey Replication. *Am J Psychiatry.* 2006;163:716-723.

5. Visser SN, Lesesne CA, Perou R. National estimates and factors associated with medication treatment for childhood attention-deficit/hyperactivity disorder. *Pediatrics.* 2007;119(Suppl 1):S99-S106.

6. Polanczyk G, de Lima MS, Horta BL, Biederman J, Rohde LA. The worldwide prevalence of ADHD: a systematic review and metaregression analysis. *Am J Psychiatry.* 2007;164:942-948.

7. Pelham WE, Foster EM, Robb JA. The economic impact of attention-deficit/hyperactivity disorder in children and adolescents. *J Pediatr Psychol.* 2007;32:711-727.

8. Spencer TJ, Biederman J, Mick E. Attention-deficit/hyperactivity disorder: diagnosis, lifespan, comorbidities, and neurobiology. *J Pediatr Psychol.* 2007;32:631-642.

9. Wilens TE, Faraone SV, Biederman J. Attention-deficit/hyperactivity disorder in adults. *JAMA.* 2004;292:619-623.

10. Faraone SV, Biederman J, Spencer T, et al. Attention-deficit/hyperactivity disorder in adults: an overview. *Biol Psychiatry.* 2000;48:9-20.

11. Biederman J, Faraone SV, Spencer TJ, Mick E, Monuteaux MC, Aleardi M. Functional impairments in adults with self-reports of diagnosed ADHD: A controlled study of 1001 adults in the community. *J Clin Psychiatry.* 2006;67:524-540.

12. Mannuzza S, Klein RG, Bessler A, Malloy P, LaPadula M. Adult outcome of hyperactive boys. Educational achievement, occupational rank, and psychiatric status. *Arch Gen Psychiatry.* 1993;50:565-576.

13. Faraone SV, Sergeant J, Gillberg C, Biederman J. The worldwide prevalence of ADHD: is it an American condition? *World Psychiatry.* 2003;2:104-113.

14. Gershon J. A meta-analytic review of gender differences in ADHD. *J Atten Disord.* 2002;5:143-154.

15. Biederman J, Faraone SV, Spencer T, Wilens T, Mick E, Lapey KA. Gender differences in a sample of adults with attention deficit hyperactivity disorder. *Psychiatry Res.* 1994;53:13-29.

16. Biederman J, Mick E, Faraone SV. Age-dependent decline of symptoms of attention deficit hyperactivity disorder: impact of remission definition and symptom type. *Am J Psychiatry.* 2000;157:816-818.

17. Lahey BB, Applegate B, McBurnett K, et al. DSM-IV field trials for attention deficit hyperactivity disorder in children and adolescents. *Am J Psychiatry.* 1994;151:1673-1685.

18. American Academy of Pediatrics. Clinical practice guideline: diagnosis and evaluation of the child with attention-deficit/hyperactivity disorder. *Pediatrics.* 2000;105:1158-1170.

19. Dulcan M. Practice parameters for the assessment and treatment of children, adolescents, and adults with attention-deficit/hyperactivity disorder. American Academy of Child and Adolescent Psychiatry. *J Am Acad Child Adolesc Psychiatry.* 1997;36(Suppl):85S-121S.

20. Applegate B, Lahey BB, Hart EL, et al. Validity of the age-of-onset criterion for ADHD: a report from the *DSM-IV* field trials. *J Am Acad Child Adolesc Psychiatry.* 1997;36:1211-1221.

21. Barkley RA, Biederman J. Toward a broader definition of the age-of-onset criterion for attention-deficit hyperactivity disorder. *J Am Acad Child Adolesc Psychiatry.* 1997;36:1204-1210.

22. Polanczyk G, Caspi A, Houts R, Kollins SH, Rohde LA, Moffitt TE. Implications of extending the ADHD age-of-onset criterion to age 12: results from a prospectively studied birth cohort. *J Am Acad Child Adolesc Psychiatry.* 2010;49:210-216.

23. Achenbach TM, Rescorla L. *Manual for the ASEBA Preschool Forms & Profiles.* Burlington, VT: University of Vermont, Research Center for Children, Youth, and Families; 2000.

24. Achenbach TM, Rescorla L. *Manual for the ASEBA School-age Forms & Profiles.* Burlington, VT: University of Vermont, Research Center for Children, Youth, and Families; 2001.

25. Ullmann RK, Sleator EK, Sprague RL, MetriTech Staff. *AD/HD Comprehensive Teacher's Rating Scale (ACTeRS).* 2nd edn. 1998 Revision. Champaign, IL: MetriTech, Inc; 1998.

26. DuPaul GJ, Power TJ, Anastopoulos AD, Reid R. *ADHD Rating Scale-IV: Checklists, Norms, and Clinical Interpretation.* New York, NY: Guilford Press; 1998.

27. Gadow KD, Sprafkin J. *ADHD Symptom Checklist-4 Manual.* Stony Brook, NY: Checkmate Plus; 1997.

28. Reynolds CR, Kamphaus RW. Behavior *Assessment System for Children, Second Edition (BASC-2) Manual.* Circle Pines, MN: AGS Publishing; 2004.

29. Brown TE. *Brown Attention Deficit Disorder Scales for Adolescents and Adults, Manual.* San Antonio, TX: The Psychological Corporation; 1996.

30. Brown TE. *Brown Attention Deficit Disorder Scales for Children and Adolescents, Manual.* San Antonio, TX: The Psychological Corporation; 2001.

31. Conners CK. *Conners 3rd Edition (Conners 3) Manual.* Toronto, ON: Multi-Health Systems, Inc; 2008.

32. Conners CK. Conners *Comprehensive Behavior Rating Scales (Conners CBRS) Manual*. Toronto, ON: Multi-Health Systems, Inc; 2008.

33. Conners CK. *Conners Early Childhood (Conners EC) Manual*. Toronto, ON: Multi-Health Systems, Inc; 2009.

34. Swanson JM. *SNAP-IV Scale*. Irvine, CA: University of California Child Development Center; 1995.

35. Wolraich ML, Lambert W, Doffing MA, Bickman L, Simmons T, Worley K. Psychometric Properties of the Vanderbilt ADHD Diagnostic Parent Rating Scale in a referred population. *J Ped Psychology*. 2003;28:559-568.

36. Wolraich ML, Feurer ID, Hannah JN, Baumgaertel A, Pinnock TY. Obtaining systematic teacher reports of disruptive behavior disorders utilizing *DSM-IV*. *J Abnorm Child Psychol*. 1998;26:141-152.

37. Sparrow EP. *Essentials of Conners Behavior Assessments*. Hoboken, NJ: John Wiley & Sons, Inc; 2010.

38. American Psychiatric Association. *Diagnostic and Statistical Manual of Mental Disorders*. 4th edn. Washington, DC: American Psychiatric Association; 1994.

39. Faries DE, Yalcin I, Harder D, Heiligenstein JH. Validation of the ADHD Rating Scale as a clinician administered and scored instrument. *J Atten Disorders*. 2001;5:107-114.

40. Zhang S, Faries DE, Vowles M, Michelson D. ADHD Rating Scale IV: psychometric properties from a multinational study as a clinician-administered instrument. *Int J Methods in Psychiatr Res*. 2005;14:186-201.

41. Power TJ, Doherty BJ, Panichelli-Mindel SM, et al. The predictive validity of parent and teacher reports of ADHD symptoms. *J Psychopathol Behav*. 1998;20:57-81.

42. DuPaul GJ, Anastopoulos AD, Power TJ, Reid R, Ikeda MJ, McGoey KE. Parent ratings of attention-deficit/hyperactivity disorder symptoms: factor structure and normative data. *J Psychopathol Behav*. 1998;20:83-102.

43. DuPaul GJ, Power TJ, Anastopoulos AD, Reid R, McGoey KE, Ikeda MJ. Teacher ratings of attention-deficit/hyperactivity disorder symptoms: factor structure and normative data. *Psychol Assessment*. 1997;9:436-444.

44. DuPaul GJ, Power TJ, McGoey KE, Ikeda MJ, Anastopoulos AD. Reliability and validity of parent and teacher ratings of attention-deficit/hyperactivity disorder symptoms. *J Psychoeduc Assess*. 1998;16:55-68.

45. Stein MA, Sarampote CS, Waldman ID, et al. A dose-response study of OROS methylphenidate in children with attention-deficit/hyperactivity disorder. *Pediatrics*. 2003;112:e404-e413.

46. Swanson J, Nolan W, Pelham WE. *SNAP Rating Scale*. Washington, DC: Educational Resources Information Center (ERIC); 1982.

47. American Psychiatric Association. *Diagnostic and Statistical Manual of Mental Disorders*. 3rd edn. Washington, DC: American Psychiatric Association; 1980.

48. American Psychiatric Association. *Diagnostic and Statistical Manual of Mental Disorders*. 3rd edn. Text revision. Washington, DC: American Psychiatric Association; 1987.

49. Loney J, Milich R. Hyperactivity, inattention, and aggression in clinical practice. In Wolraich M, Routh D, eds. *Advances in Developmental and Behavioral Pediatrics*. Greenwich, CT: JAI; 1982:113-147.

50. Murray DW, Bussing R, Fernandez M, et al. Psychometric properties of teacher SKAMP ratings from a community sample. *Assessment*. 2009;16:193-208.

51. Bussing R, Fernandez M, Harwood M, et al. Parent and teacher SNAP-IV ratings of attention deficit hyperactivity disorder symptoms: psychometric properties and normative ratings from a school district sample. *Assessment*. 2008;15:317-328.

52. Swanson J, Schuck S, Mann M, et al. Categorical and dimensional definitions and evaluations of symptoms of ADHD: the SNAP and SWAN rating scales. http://ADHD.net. adhd.net. 2001. 2010. Accessed November 18, 2010.

53. Steele M, Weiss M, Swanson J, Wang J, Prinzo RS, Binder CE. A randomized, controlled, effectiveness trial of oros-methylphenidate compared to usual care with immediate-release methylphenidate in attention deficit-hyperactivity disorder. *Can J Clin Pharmacol*. 2006;13:e50-e62.

54. Dell'Agnello G, Maschietto D, Bravaccio C, et al. Atomoxetine hydrochloride in the treatment of children and adolescents with attention-deficit/hyperactivity disorder and comorbid oppositional defiant disorder: A placebo-controlled Italian study. *Eur Neuropsychopharmacol*. 2009;19:822–834.

55. Wigal SB, Steinhoff K, McGough JJ, et al. St.A.R.T.: Strattera/Adderall XR randomized trial. Presented at: *17th Annual US Psychiatric and Mental Health Congress*; November 19, 2004; San Diego, CA. Poster Presentation 64.

56. Sprafkin J, Gadow KD, Nolan EE. The utility of a DSM-IV-referenced screening instrument for attention-deficit/hyperactivity disorder. *J Emotional Behav Dis*. 2001;9:182-191.

57. Gadow KD, Nolan EE, Sverd J, Sprafkin J, Paolicelli L. Methylphenidate in aggressive-hyperactive boys: I. Effects on peer aggression in public school settings. *J Am Acad Child Adolesc Psychiatry*. 1990;29:710-778.

58. Sprafkin J, Gadow KD. Choosing an attention-deficit/hyperactivity disorder rating scale: is item randomization necessary? *J Child Adolesc Psychopharmacol*. 2007;17:75-84.

59. Rucklidge JJ, Tannock R. Validity of the Brown ADD scales: An investigation in a predominantly inattentive ADHD adolescent sample with and without reading disabilities. *J Atten Disord*. 2002;5:155-164.

60. Reynolds CR, Kamphaus RW. *Behavior Assessment System for Children (BASC) Manual*. Circle Pines, MN: AGS Publishing; 1992.

61. Achenbach TM, Rescorla L. *Manual for the ASEBA Adult Forms and Profiles*. Burlington, VT: University of Vermont, Research Center for Children, Youth, and Families; 2003.

62. Achenbach TM, Newhouse PA, Rescorla L. *Manual for the ASEBA Older Adult Forms and Profiles.* Burlington, VT: University of Vermont, Research Center for Children, Youth, and Families; 2004.

63. Achenbach TM, Rescorla L. *Multicultural Supplement to the Manual for the ASEBA School-age Forms and Profiles.* Burlington, VT: University of Vermont, Research Center for Children, Youth, and Families; 2007.

64. Kessler RC, Adler L, Ames M, et al. The World Health Organization Adult ADHD Self-Report Scale (ASRS): a short screening scale for use in the general population. *Psychol Med.* 2005;35:245-256.

65. Spencer TJ, Adler LA, Qiao M, et al. Validation of the Adult ADHD Investigator Symptom Rating Scale (AISRS). *J Atten Disord.* 2010;14:57-68.

66. Conners C, Erhardt D, Sparrow E, MHS Staff. *The Conners Adult ADHD Rating Scale (CAARS).* Toronto, ON: Multi-Health Systems, Inc; 1998.

67. Ward MF, Wender PH, Reimherr FW. The Wender Utah Rating Scale: an aid in the retrospective diagnosis of childhood attention deficit hyperactivity disorder. *Am J Psychiatry.* 1993;150:885-890.

68. Adler LA, Goodman DW, Kollins SH, et al. Double-blind, placebo-controlled study of the efficacy and safety of lisdexamfetamine dimesylate in adults with attention-deficit/hyperactivity disorder. *J Clin Psychiatry.* 2008;69:1364-1373.

69. Adler LA, Spencer T, Faraone SV, et al. Training raters to assess adult ADHD: reliability of ratings. *J Atten Disord.* 2005;8:121-126.

70. Adler LA, Spencer T, Faraone SV, et al. Validity of pilot Adult ADHD Self- Report Scale (ASRS) to rate adult ADHD symptoms. *Ann Clin Psychiatry.* 2006;18:145-148.

71. Kessler RC, Adler LA, Gruber MJ, Sarawate CA, Spencer T, Van Brunt DL. Validity of the World Health Organization Adult ADHD Self-Report Scale (ASRS) Screener in a representative sample of health plan members. *Int J Methods Psychiatr Res.* 2007;16:52-65.

72. Landgraf JM, Rich M, Rappaport L. Measuring quality of life in children with attention-deficit/hyperactivity disorder and their families. *Arch Pediatr Adolesc Med.* 2002;156:384-391.

73. Adler LA, Spencer T, Brown TE, et al. Once-daily atomoxetine for adult attention-deficit/hyperactivity disorder: a 6-month, double-blind trial. *J Clin Psychopharmacol.* 2009;29:44-50.

74. Biederman J, Mick E, Spencer T, et al. An open-label trial of OROS methylphenidate in adults with late-onset ADHD. *CNS Spectr.* 2006;11:390-396.

75. Solanto, MV, Marks AJ, Mitchell KJ, Wasserstein J, Kofman MD. Development of a new psychosocial treatment for adult ADHD. *J Atten Disord.* 2008;11:728-736.

76. Virta M, Vedenpää A, Grönroos N, et al. Adults with ADHD benefit from cognitive-behaviorally oriented group rehabilitation: a study of 29 participants. *J Atten Disord.* 2008;12:218-226.

77. Adler LA, Spencer TJ, Milton DR, Moore RJ, Michelson D. Long-term, open-label study of the safety and efficacy of atomoxetine in adults with attention-deficit/hyperactivity disorder: an interim analysis. *J Clin Psychiatry.* 2005;66:294-299.

78. Durell T, Adler L, Wilens T, Paczkowski M, Schuh K. Atomoxetine treatment for ADHD: younger adults compared with older adults. *J Atten Disord*. 2010;13:401-406.

79. Rossini ED, O'Connor MA. Retrospective self-reported symptoms of attention-deficit hyperactivity disorder: reliability of the Wender Utah Rating Scale. *Psychol Rep*. 1995;77:751-754.

80. Stein MA, Sandoval R, Szumowski E, et al. Psychometric characteristics of the Wender Utah Rating Scale (WURS): reliability and factor structure for men and women. *Psychopharmacol Bull*. 1995;31:425-433.

81. Landgraf JM. Monitoring quality of life in adults with ADHD: reliability and validity of a new measure. *J Atten Disord*. 2007;11:351-362.

82. Brod M, Johnston J, Able S, Swindle R. Validation of the adult attention-deficit/hyperactivity disorder quality-of-life Scale (AAQoL): a disease-specific quality-of-life measure. *Qual Life Res*. 2006;15:117-129.

83. Starfield B, Bergner M, Ensminger M, Riley AW, Green BF, Ryan S. *Child Health and Illness Profile-Adolescent Edition (CHIP-AE)*. Baltimore, MD: The Johns Hopkins University; 1994.

84. Riley AW, Forrest C, Starfield B, Rebok G, Green B, Robertson J. *Child Health and Illness Profile-Child Edition (CHIP-CE)*. Baltimore, MD: The Johns Hopkins University; 2001.

85. Landgraf JM, Abetz L, Ware JE. *The CHQ User's Manual*. 2nd Printing. Boston, MA: HealthAct; 1999.

86. Varni JW, Seid M, Kurtin PS. PedsQL™ 4.0: Reliability and validity of the Pediatric Quality of Life Inventory™ Version 4.0 Generic Core Scales in healthy and patient populations. Medical Care. 2001;39:800-812.

87. Weiss MD, Wasdell MB, Bomben MM. Weiss Functional Impairment Rating Scale—Parent Report (WFIRS-P). BC Children's Hospital. http://bcchildrens.ca/NR/rdonlyres/F6C1AD32-CF47-47A7-AE97-F37FDF850DC4/20927/WFIRSParentReport.pdf. November 29, 2004. Accessed November 18, 2010.

88. Weiss MD. Weiss Functional Impairment Rating Scale Self-Report (WFIRS-S). Adult ADHD NACE Toolkit Assessment Tools, University of British Columbia. www.naceonline.com/AdultADHDtoolkit/assessmenttools/wfirs.pdf. 2000. September 20, 2010.

89. Patrick DL, Edwards TC, Topolski TD. Adolescent quality of life, part II: Initial validation of a new instrument. *J Adolesce*. 2002;25:287-300.

90. Harpin VA. The effect of ADHD on the life of an individual, their family, and community from preschool to adult life. *Arch Dis Child*. 2005;90:i2-i7.

91. Escobar R, Soutullo CA, Hervas A, et al. Worse quality of life for children with newly diagnosed attention-deficit/hyperactivity disorder, compared with asthmatic and healthy children. *Pediatrics*. 2005;116:e364-e369.

92. Varni JW, Burwinkle TM. The PedsQL™ as a patient-reported outcome in children and adolescents with attention-deficit/hyperactivity disorder. Health Qual Life Outcomes. 2006;4:1-10.

93. Klassen AF, Miller A, Fine S. Health-related quality of life in children and adolescents who have a diagnosis of attention-deficit/hyperactivity disorder. *Pediatrics*. 2004;114:e541-e547.

94. Wong ICK, Asherson P, Bilbow A, et al. Cessation of attention deficit hyperactivity disorder drugs in the young (CADDY) – a pharmacoepidemiological and qualitative study. *Health Technol Assesst*. 2009;13:iii-x,ix-xi,1-120.

95. Food and Drug Administration (FDA). *Guidance for Industry: Patient-reported Outcome Measures: Use in Medical Product Development to Support Labeling Claims*. Rockville, MD: FDA; 2009.

96. Committee for Medicinal Products for Human Use. Reflection paper on the regulatory guidance for the use of health related quality of life (HRQL) measures in the evaluation of medicinal products. www.emea.europa.eu/docs/en_GB/document_library/Scientific_guideline/2009/09/WC500003637.pdf. July 27, 2005. Accessed November 18, 2010.

97. Bukstein O, Arnold LE, Landgraf J, Hodgkins P. Does switching from oral extended-release methylphenidate to the methylphenidate transdermal system affect health-related quality-of-life and medication satisfaction for children with attention-deficit/hyperactivity disorder? *Child Adolesc Psychiatry and Ment Health*. 2009;3:39-50.

98. Spencer TJ, Adler LA, Weisler RH, Youcha SH. Triple-bead mixed amphetamine salts (SPD465), a novel, enhanced extended-release amphetamine formulation for the treatment of adults with ADHD: a randomized, double-blind, multicenter, placebo-controlled study. *J Clin Psychiatry*. 2008;69:1437-1448.

99. Spencer TJ, Landgraf JM, Adler LA, Weisler RH, Anderson CS, Youcha SH. Attention-deficit/hyperactivity disorder-specific quality of life with triple-bead mixed amphetamine salts (SPD465) in adults: results of a randomized, double-blind, placebo-controlled study. *J Clin Psychiatry*. 2008;69:1766-1775.

100. Matza LS, Johnston JA, Faries DE, Malley KG, Brod M. Responsiveness of the Adult Attention-Deficit/Hyperactivity Disorder Quality of Life Scale (AAQoL). *Qual Life Res*. 2007;16:1511-1520.

101. Riley AW, Coghill D, Forrest CB, et al; for the ADORE Study Group. Validity of the health-related quality of life assessment in the ADORE study: parent report form of the CHIP-Child Edition. *Eur Child Adolesc Psychiatry*. 2006;15(Suppl 1):i63-i71.

102. Riley AW, Forrest CB, Rebok GW, et al. The child report form of the CHIP-Child Edition: reliability and validity. *Med Care*. 2004;42:221-231.

103. Riley AW, Forrest CB, Starfield B, Rebok GW, Robertson JA, Green BF. The parent report form of the CHIP-Child Edition: reliability and validity. *Med Care*. 2004;42:210-220.

104. Escobar R, Schacht A, Wehmeier PM, Wagner T. Quality of life and attention-deficit/hyperactivity disorder core symptoms: a pooled analysis of 5 non-US atomoxetine clinical trials. *J Clin Psychopharmacol*. 2010;30:145-151.

105. Starfield B, Riley AW, Green BF, et al. The adolescent child health and illness profile. A population-based measure of health. *Med Care*. 1995;33:553-566.

106. Riley AW, Forrest CB, Starfield B, Green B, Kang M, Ensminger M. Reliability and validity of the adolescent health profile-types. *Med Care*. 1998;36:1237-1248.

107. Perwien AR, Faries DE, Kratochvil CJ, Sumner CR, Kelsey DK, Allen AJ. Improvement in Health-Related Quality of Life in Children with ADHD: an analysis of placebo controlled studies of atomoxetine. *J Dev Behav Pediatr*. 2004;25:264-271.

108. Varni JW, Burwinkle TM, Seid M. The PedsQL™ as a pediatric patient-reported outcome: reliability and validity of the PedsQL™ measurement model in 25,000 children. *Expert Rev Pharmacoecon Outcomes Res*. 2005;5:705-719.

109. Varni JW, Limbers CA, Burwinkle TM. Parent proxy-report of their children's health-related quality of life: An analysis of 13,878 parents' reliability and validity across age subgroups using the PedsQL™ 4.0 Generic Core Scales. *Health Qual Life Outcomes*. 2007;5:2.

110. Limbers CA, Ripperger-Suhler J, Boutton K, Ransom D, Varni JW. A comparative analysis of health-related quality of life and family impact between children with ADHD treated in a general pediatric clinic and a psychiatric clinic utilizing the PedsQL. *J Atten Disord*. January 11, 2010. [Epub ahead of print].

111. Maziade M, Rouleau N, Lee B, Rogers A, Davis L, Dickson R. Atomoxetine and neuropsychological function in children with attention-deficit/hyperactivity disorder: results of a pilot study. *J Child Adolesc Psychopharmacol*. 2009;19:709-718.

112. Topolski TD, Edwards TC, Patrick DL, Varley P, Way ME Buesching DP. Quality of life of adolescent males with attention-deficit hyperactivity disorder. *J Atten Disord*. 2004;7:163-173.

113. Conners CK, March JM. *Conners–March Developmental Questionnaire*. North Tonowanda, NY: Multi-Health Systems, Inc; 1999.

114. Shaffer D, Fisher P, Lucas CP, Dulcan MK, Schwab-Stone ME. NIMH Diagnostic Interview Schedule for Children Version IV (DISC-IV): description, differences from previous versions, and reliability of some common diagnoses. *J Am Acad Child and Adolesc Psychiatry*. 2000;39:28-38.

115. Reich W, Welner Z, Herjanic B, MHS Staff. *Diagnostic Interview for Children and Adolescents-IV (DICA-IV)*. North Tonowanda, NY: Multi-Health Systems, Inc; 1997.

116. Kaufman J, Birmaher B, Brent D, Rao U, Ryan N. *Schedule for Affective Disorders and Schizophrenia for School-Age Children, Present and Lifetime Version (K-SADS-PL)*. Pittsburgh, PA: Department of Psychiatry, University of Pittsburgh School of Medicine; 1996.

117. Lewczyk CM, Garland AF, Hurlburt MS, Gearity J, Hough RL. Comparing DISC-IV and clinician diagnoses among youths receiving public mental health services. *J Am Acad Child Adolesc Psychiatry*. 2003;42:349-56.

118. Reich W. Diagnostic interview for children and adolescents (DICA). *J Am Acad Child Adolesc Psychiatry*. 2000;39:59-66.

119. Birmaher B, Ehmann M, Axelson DA, et al. Schedule for affective disorders and schizophrenia for school-age children (K-SADS-PL) for the assessment of preschool children–a preliminary psychometric study. *J Psychiatr Res*. 2009;43:680-686.

120. Kaufman J, Birmaher B, Brent D, et al. Schedule for Affective Disorders and Schizophrenia for School-Age Children-Present and Lifetime Version (K-SADS-PL): initial reliability and validity data. *J Am Acad Child Adolesc Psychiatry.* 1997;36:980-988.

121. Adler L, Spencer T. *The Adult ADHD Clinical Diagnostic Scale (ACDS) V 1.2.* New York, NY: University School of Medicine; 2004.

122. Epstein JN, Johnson D, Conners CK. *Conners' Adult ADHD Diagnostic Interview for DSM-IV.* North Tonawanda, NY: Multi-Health Systems, Inc; 2000.

123. Adler L, Cohen J. Diagnosis and evaluation of adults with attention-deficit/hyperactivity disorder. *Psychiatr Clin North Am.* 2004;27:187-201.

124. Michelson D, Adler L, Spencer T, et al. Atomoxetine in adults with ADHD: two randomized, placebo-controlled studies. *Biol Psychiatry.* 2003;53:112-120.

125. Spencer T, Biederman J, Wilens T, et al. Efficacy of a mixed amphetamine salts compound in adults with attention-deficit/hyperactivity disorder. *Arch Gen Psychiatry.* 2001;58:775-782.

126. Epstein JN, Kollins SH. Psychometric properties of an adult ADHD diagnostic interview. *J Atten Disord.* 2006;9:504-514.

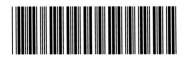